*Self Care Hygiene **2023 Edition***

Feminine
Intimate Care

Guide and Tips To Maintaining Intimate Hygiene & Freshness

By **CYNTHIA LEONARD**

INTRODUCTION: **5**

Understanding Feminine Intimate Care   5

The Importance of Feminine Intimate Care   6

Common Myths and Misconceptions   7

FEMALE ANATOMY AND PHYSIOLOGY   **8**

Exploring Female Reproductive Anatomy   8

External Anatomy: Vulva and Labia   9

Internal Anatomy: Vagina, Cervix and Uterus   10

HORMONAL CHANGES AND THE MENSTRUAL CYCLE   **11**

Menstruation: Normal Processes and Challenges   12

Managing Menstrual Health and Comfort   13

MAINTAINING FEMININE HYGIENE   **15**

Essential Hygiene Practices and Daily Hygiene Routine   15

Proper Cleansing Techniques   16

Choosing the Right Intimate Care Products   17

THE IMPORTANCE OF PH BALANCE   **19**

Understanding pH and Its Impact   19

Maintaining Optimal Vaginal pH   20

pH-Balanced Products and Their Benefits   21

MANAGING ODOUR AND DISCHARGE   **23**

Normal vs. Abnormal Odour and Discharge   23

Tips for Managing Odour and Discharge   24

Natural Remedies and Lifestyle Changes   25

NURTURING INTIMATE WELLNESS   **27**

Maintaining Vaginal Health   27

Preventing Infections: Yeast, Bacterial Vaginosis, and UTIs   28

Addressing Common Vaginal Issues   29

More Typical Vaginal Problems and Advice on How to Treat Them: 30

Vaginal Health at Different Stages of Life   31

SEXUAL WELLNESS AND INTIMACY   **33**

Sexual Health Education   33

Communicating with Partners about Intimate Care   35

Safe Sex Practices and Protection: Postpartum Care and Recovery 38

    Understanding the Changes After Pregnancy 40

    Nurturing Physical and Emotional Recovery 42

    Caring for the Pelvic Floor 45

HOLISTIC APPROACHES TO FEMININE CARE **47**

    Diet and Nutrition for Feminine Health 47

    Nourishing Foods for Hormonal Balance 50

    Nutrients for Optimal Vaginal Health 52

EXERCISE AND FITNESS FOR THE PELVIC FLOOR **54**

    Strengthening Pelvic Floor Muscles 54

    Recommended Exercises and Techniques for Women 57

FEMININE CARE: STRESS MANAGEMENT AND EMOTIONAL WELL-BEING **60**

THE MIND-BODY CONNECTION **63**

STRATEGIES FOR STRESS REDUCTION **66**

SELF-CARE AND EMOTIONAL SUPPORT **70**

CONCLUSION: **73**

    Embracing Feminine Intimate Care 73

INTRODUCTION:

Understanding Feminine Intimate Care

The practices and goods used to preserve the comfort, cleanliness and health of the female genital region are referred to as feminine intimate care. It encompasses a variety of personal hygiene practices and decisions that support wellbeing and guard against possible problems including infections, irritability and discomfort. To preserve their overall reproductive health, women must learn and put into practise proper feminine intimate care. Here are some important factors to think about:

Gentle Cleaning: It's crucial to frequently clean the external genital region using hypoallergenic, fragrance-free, pH-balanced cleansers made especially for intimate use. The natural pH balance in the region might be upset by using strong soaps, douches or scented items, which can irritate the delicate skin nearby.

Correct Wiping Technique: To avoid germs from the anal region entering the urethra and vagina, which may cause urinary tract infections, always remember to wipe from front to back while using the toilet.

Menstrual Hygiene: To reduce the risk of infections and bacterial overgrowth during menstruation, it is essential to replace sanitary pads, tampons, or menstrual cups often *(usually every 4 to 8 hours)*. Select items that are cosy and appropriate for your flow.

Breathable Underwear: Wear breathable pants to keep your genital region dry and avoid the development of germs and fungus. Choose pants made of breathable materials like cotton. Avoid wearing synthetic fabrics or tight-fitting pants for long periods of time since they might trap moisture and raise the possibility of discomfort.

Be Careful not to Overwash: While it is important to keep the genital region clean, overwashing or using too many powerful cleaners may upset the natural balance of bacteria and moisture, resulting in dryness, irritability, or infections. Avoid harsh scrubbing and stick to soft cleaning.

Diet and Hydration: Staying well hydrated is good for many aspects of health, including the vaginal region. The body can stay hydrated and maintain healthy vaginal secretions by drinking enough water. A healthy diet that emphasises fruits, vegetables, and probiotics may also promote vaginal health.

Regular Check-ups: Regular check-ups are essential for keeping track of reproductive health, seeing any problems before they become serious and getting expert advice on personal care.

Every woman's body is different, so it's crucial to pay attention to what yours requires and feels comfortable with. Consult a healthcare provider for the best guidance and care if you have ongoing pain, odd discharge, itching or any other unsettling symptoms.

The Importance of Feminine Intimate Care

The issue of feminine intimate care is very important and is crucial for women's general health and wellbeing. Here are some major justifications for why female intimate care is essential:

Promoting Hygiene: In order to avoid the growth of bacteria, yeast, and other germs that may cause illnesses such as urinary tract infections (UTIs), yeast infections and bacterial vaginosis, proper hygiene is essential. Regular washing with gentle, pH-balanced cleansers helps maintain cleanliness and lowers the risk of infections in the external genital region.

Preventing Irritation and Pain: The genital region is delicate and poor care may lead to discomfort, itching, dryness or irritation. The natural pH balance, moisture levels and general comfort of the region are maintained by using mild, fragrance-free products made especially for intimate use.

Supporting Vaginal Health: Maintaining the natural balance of healthy bacteria is essential for vaginal health since the vagina has its own self-cleaning system. This equilibrium may be upset by harsh soaps, douching or excessive cleaning, which can result in imbalances, infections or bad odours. A healthy vaginal environment may be supported by using products that are mild and specially made for the intimate region.

Managing Menstrual Hygiene: Taking care of menstrual hygiene is important for both infection prevention and comfort during the period. Regularly replacing sanitary items like pads, tampons, or menstrual cups aids in maintaining cleanliness and halts the formation of germs.

Increasing Self-Confidence: Taking good care of one's intimate region may help a lady feel more confident and self-assured in general. Women may carry out their everyday tasks with a feeling of well-being when they feel clean, fresh and comfy.

Every woman should use caution while providing personal care. The natural equilibrium of the vagina may be upset by excessive washing, harsh detergents or douching, which raises the risk of infections.

Common Myths and Misconceptions

There are several widespread misunderstandings and fallacies about feminine intimate care. To name a few:

Myth: To maintain a healthy vagina, feminine hygiene products are required.
In actuality, the vagina cleans itself and doesn't need feminine hygiene items like douches or scented soaps. Using such items may cause discomfort or infections by upsetting the normal balance of microorganisms in the vagina. Most of the time, gentle washing with warm water suffices.

Myth: In order to keep clean, pubic hair must be waxed or shaved.
Reality: By acting as a barrier to protect the vaginal region, pubic hair has a useful function. Pubic hair removal is a matter of personal preference and has no effect on hygiene. Maintaining genital cleanliness is more essential than proper hygiene, including routine washing.

Myth: Vaginal odours are unusual and need to be covered up.
In actuality, the odour of the vagina varies based on things including food, hormones and general health. Mild odour changes are often normal and not reason for alarm. Strong, unpleasant or fishy smells may be signs of an illness and should be assessed by a medical practitioner rather than covered up with fragrances or sprays.

Myth: Vaginas should always look a specific way or be tight.
There is no one "normal" or "ideal " to look for a vagina in terms of size, shape or colour. The idea that a vagina should be tight or have certain qualities is often founded on erroneous cultural norms. Because everybody is different, natural deviations are quite normal.

Myth: Natural components are always safe to use in feminine hygiene products.
Reality: The use of natural substances does not always imply safety. Some organic materials, including some plant extracts or essential oils, might irritate or trigger allergic responses in people with sensitive skin. If you have questions about a product's safety or effectiveness, it's vital to read the label, do some research and talk to a doctor.

To provide correct information and support healthy practices when it comes to feminine intimate care, it's critical to dispel these myths and misunderstandings.

FEMALE ANATOMY AND PHYSIOLOGY

Exploring Female Reproductive Anatomy

The tissues and organs involved in the female reproductive process are referred to as female reproductive anatomy. These organs are in charge of egg formation, fertilisation, pregnancy and delivery. Investigating the key elements of the female reproductive system is as follows:

Ovaries: On each side of the uterus are two tiny, almond-shaped structures known as the ovaries. They go through a procedure called ovulation to generate and release eggs (ova). Hormones like progesterone and oestrogen are also produced by the ovaries.

Fallopian Tubes: The fallopian tubes, often called uterine tubes or oviducts, join the ovaries to the uterus. They provide the eggs with a route from the ovaries to the uterus. A sperm and an egg are normally fertilised within the fallopian tubes.

Uterus: During pregnancy, a fertilised egg implants and grows into a foetus in the uterus, also known as the womb. It is separated into two major sections: the body, which is the top portion and the cervix, which is the bottom portion. Throughout the menstrual cycle, the uterus goes through monthly cycles of lining thickening and shedding.

Cervix: The cervix, which links the uterus to the vagina, is the lowest, thin portion of the organ. It has a little gap, known as the cervical os, through which menstrual blood may flow from the uterus into the vagina. The cervix widens during delivery to provide room for the baby to pass through.

Vagina: The muscular channel known as the vagina runs from the cervix to the external genitalia. It functions as the birth canal during delivery and accepts the penis during sex. Numerous creases and stretchy tissue in the vaginal walls allow for both delivery and sexual activity.

Vulva: External female genitalia are referred to as the vulva. The clitoris, a highly sensitive organ linked to sexual pleasure, the labia majora and minora, the urethral entrance and the vaginal opening are all included in this region.

Mammary Glands: Breasts or mammary glands, have a role in reproduction via nursing even though they are not a direct component of the reproductive system. After giving birth, they make milk to feed the baby.

The ovulation, fertilisation, implantation, pregnancy and birthing processes in females are made easier by the cooperation of these tissues. It's important to note that although the overall form and functions of a woman's reproductive anatomy may vary from person to person.

External Anatomy: Vulva and Labia

The female reproductive system's external genitalia are known as the vulva. It contains a number of components, including the clitoris, labia majora, labia minora and the vaginal entrance, which is situated between the legs. Let's examine each of these structures in more detail:

Labia Majora: The vulva's outermost folds are known as the labia majora. They often have fat deposits and are meaty, protecting the vulva's other components. The labia minora, clitoris, vaginal entrance and urethral opening are enclosed and protected by them. Usually, the labia majora are bigger and more noticeable than the labia minora.

Labia Minora: The labia minora are the vulva's tiny inner folds. They may vary in size, shape and colour amongst people and they are located inside the labia majora. The labia minora may stay inside the folds of the labia majora or protrude outside of them. They are abundant in blood arteries and have many sebaceous glands.

Clitoris: At the anterior intersection of the labia minora is the clitoris, a highly sensitive and sexually responsive organ. The clitoral hood, a hood of skin, often covers it. The clitoris has a glans, a shaft and erectile tissue, which are anatomically identical to the penis. It is essential to arousal and pleasure during sexual activity.

Vaginal Opening: The introitus, sometimes referred to as the vaginal opening, is the opening to the vagina. The hymen, a thin membrane that may partly enclose or cover the aperture, is usually partially covering it; it is situated between the labia minora. The vaginal opening enables menstrual blood to flow through as well as sexual activity and birthing.

Do note that each person might have a drastically different vulva in terms of size and appearance. This regular natural fluctuation does not portend any health issues.

Internal Anatomy: Vagina, Cervix and Uterus

Vagina:

A muscular channel called the vagina is part of the female reproductive system. It reaches all the way to the cervix from the vulva *(external genitalia)*. The vagina is used for menstrual flow as well as sexual activity, childbirth and other processes.

Cervix:

The cervix, which links the vagina to the higher reproductive organs, is the lowest portion of the uterus. The cervical os is a cylindrical or conical structure with a little hole. In order to keep the female reproductive system healthy, the cervix is essential. During the menstrual cycle, it generates mucus that fluctuates in consistency, enabling or impeding sperm from passing past the cervix.

Uterus:

The uterus, sometimes referred to as the womb, is a pear-shaped, hollow organ that is situated in the pelvic cavity between the bladder and the rectum. During pregnancy, it is principally in charge of nourishing and sustaining the growing foetus. The uterus is made up of three layers: the perimetrium, the myometrium, which is formed of smooth muscle and the endometrium, which is the innermost layer. During the menstrual cycle, the uterus goes through cyclical changes and if fertilisation does not take place, the endometrium is shed.

HORMONAL CHANGES AND THE MENSTRUAL CYCLE

The menstrual cycle, which is the monthly process experienced by women of reproductive age, is greatly influenced by hormonal changes. A complex interaction of hormones controls the uterine lining's development and shedding as well as the maturation and release of eggs from the ovaries, regulating the menstrual cycle. Although each person's menstrual cycle is unique in terms of its precise length and features, the hormonal changes often follow a predictable pattern.

The following hormones have a major role in the menstrual cycle:

Follicle-Stimulating Hormone *(FSH)***:** The pituitary gland in the brain releases FSH at the start of the cycle. In the ovaries, FSH promotes the development of follicles that each house one immature egg.

Oestrogen: As the follicles develop, they release oestrogen, which is what causes the endometrium, or uterine lining, to thicken. In addition to inhibiting the production of FSH, oestrogen also stops uncontrollable follicle development.

Luteinizing Hormone *(LH)***:** As oestrogen levels grow, the pituitary gland finally releases an increase in LH. The release of a mature egg from one of the ovaries is called ovulation and the LH surge accelerates this process.

Progesterone: Progesterone is produced by the corpus luteum, a tissue that develops from the burst follicle after ovulation. By further thickening the endometrium, progesterone aids in preparing the uterus for potential implantation of a fertilised egg.

Gonadotropin-Releasing Hormone *(GnRH)***:** GnRH, which is produced by the brain's hypothalamus and controls the pituitary gland's production of FSH and LH, is a hormone. Throughout the cycle, GnRH, FSH and LH levels change.

The corpus luteum gradually deteriorates in the absence of fertilisation, which lowers progesterone and oestrogen levels. Menstruation results from this dip, which also causes the uterine lining to shed, restarting the cycle.

The hormonal changes that occur throughout the menstrual cycle might differ from person to person and may be impacted by things like stress, nutrition, exercise and certain medical problems. Consult with a healthcare provider so they can provide you individualised advice if you have any particular queries or concerns regarding your menstrual period.

Menstruation: Normal Processes and Challenges

In the female reproductive system, menstruation is a normal phenomenon. It entails the uterine lining lost each month, which is followed by hormonal changes and bleeding. Menstruation might bring some difficulties even though it is a natural and necessary aspect of a woman's reproductive health. Let's examine both the regular procedures and difficulties related to menstruation.

Typical Procedures:

Menstrual Cycle: Although it may vary from person to person, the menstrual cycle is a cyclical event that normally lasts around 28 days. It entails preparing the uterus for a prospective pregnancy. The three stages of the cycle are the follicular phase, ovulation and luteal phase.
The first day of menstruation marks the start of the follicular phase. The ovarian follicles, which each contain an egg, are induced to expand by the hormones luteinizing hormone (LH) and follicle-stimulating hormone (FSH).

Ovulation: One developed egg is discharged from the ovary at around the 14th day of a 28-day cycle, which is the midpoint of the cycle. Ovulation is the name for this process.

Follicular Phase: Following ovulation, the burst follicle develops into the corpus luteum, which releases progesterone. This hormone primes the uterus for prospective fertilisation and implantation of an egg.

Menstruation: The corpus luteum disintegrates, hormone levels decline and the uterine lining is shed via the vagina if fertilisation is unsuccessful. The result of this shedding is menstruation, which may continue anywhere from a few days to a week. Uterine lining and blood arteries are mixed together in the blood and tissue that are purged during menstruation.

Challenges:

Menstrual cramps, also known as dysmenorrhea, are painful and uncomfortable for many women. From moderate to severe, these cramps may be accompanied by backaches, headaches and weariness. Other discomforts are also typical, including bloating, breast soreness and mood changes.

Premenstrual Syndrome (PMS): The term "premenstrual syndrome" *(PMS)* refers to a collection of emotional and physical symptoms that manifest in the days before a period. Mood swings, anger, breast tenderness, bloating, exhaustion and cravings for food are among symptoms. While moderate for some people, PMS may be really severe and have a big influence on daily life.

Heavy or Irregular Menstrual Bleeding: Menstrual bleeding that is excessive or irregular may cause anaemia, exhaustion and disruptions to everyday activities in certain women. This condition is known as menorrhagia. Others, however, could have irregular menstruation, including fluctuations in cycle length or skipped periods, which can make it difficult to forecast and prepare.

Premenstrual Dysphoric Disorder *(PMDD)* is a severe type of premenstrual syndrome *(PMS)* that affects a tiny proportion of women. It causes severe melancholy, anxiety and mood swings and has powerful emotional and physical symptoms that may seriously interrupt everyday living.

Hormonal Imbalances and Disorders: Conditions like endometriosis or polycystic ovarian syndrome *(PCOS)* that affect hormone levels may affect menstruation. These diseases may result in painful flare-ups, painful periods, problems with fertility, and other difficulties.

Stigma and Cultural Challenges: Menstruation is associated with shame, beliefs and cultural challenges in various societies. This may result in embarrassment, restricted access to hygiene supplies, insufficient menstruation knowledge and limitations on daily activities.

Even while menstruation might be difficult, it is still an essential part of reproductive health, it is crucial to remember.

Managing Menstrual Health and Comfort

Managing menstrual health and comfort is crucial to a person's overall wellbeing if they menstruate. To promote excellent menstrual health and increase comfort during this time, there are various different things you may do. The following advice:

Period Hygiene Goods: Pick period hygiene items that are comfortable for you and meet your requirements. Period knickers, tampons, menstrual cups and disposable pads are available options. Try out several items to see which ones work best for you.

Change Regularly: No matter what kind of product you use, it's essential to replace it often to preserve cleanliness and stop leaks. Change your pad or tampon every 4-6 hours or as necessary, or according to the manufacturer's recommendations.

Comfortable Attire: While on your period, dress in loose, breathable clothes. Wearing comfortable, loose-fitting clothing made of natural materials like cotton helps keep you cool and ease pain.

Pain Control: If you have period cramps, you should think about using an over-the-counter pain killer such as ibuprofen or naproxen. Another way to feel better is to use a heating pad or take a warm bath.

Stay Hydrated: Keep your body hydrated to aid with menstruation symptoms. Drinking plenty of water may also help with bloating reduction.

Balanced Diet: A well-balanced diet that includes plenty of fruits, vegetables, whole grains and lean meats will promote general health and perhaps lessen menstruation pain.

Regular Exercise: Exercise on a regular basis will help you feel better mentally, less stressed and have less menstruation symptoms. Pick enjoyable exercises like walking, running, yoga or swimming.

Controlling Stress: Stress might make menstruation symptoms worse. To help you feel less stressed during your period, try stress-relieving methods like deep breathing, meditation or participating in your favourite pastimes.

Track Your Cycle: Calendar or a period tracking software may be used to keep tabs on your menstrual cycle. By knowing when your period will arrive, you may plan properly.

Seek Medical Counsel: It's important to speak with a healthcare provider for direction and advice if you have questions about your menstrual health, are in excruciating pain or have noticed any anomalies in your cycle.

MAINTAINING FEMININE HYGIENE

Essential Hygiene Practices and Daily Hygiene Routine

For women's health and wellbeing, maintaining good cleanliness for feminine intimate care is essential. Following these basic hygiene rules can help you stay healthy:

Wash Your Hands: Before touching your intimate region, always start by properly cleansing your hands with soap and water. By doing this, the spread of bacteria and other pathogens is reduced.

Use Gentle, PH-balanced Cleansers: Stay away from harsh soaps, scented items and douches for the vaginal region. Instead, use gentle, pH-balanced cleansers designed especially for intimate use. By preserving the vagina's natural pH balance, these products lessen discomfort.

Gently Wash the Vulva: Which is the exterior genital region, while cleaning your intimate area. Gently clean the area with warm water and a tiny bit of the gentle cleaner. Abrasive materials like sponges or cloths should not be used, since they might irritate skin.

Avoid Douching: Douching should be avoided since it includes washing the vagina with water or other solutions, which might disturb the pH and microbial balance there. It is unnecessary and raises the possibility of infections and other problems. The vagina cleans itself and doesn't need to be doused.

Pat Dry After Washing: Following a thorough cleaning, pat your intimate region dry with a fresh towel. Avoid rubbing too hard since it could irritate the skin. It's crucial to make sure the area is thoroughly dry since moisture might encourage the development of germs.

Choose Breathable Undergarments: This enables air to circulate, such as cotton or other natural fibres. Avoid wearing undergarments that are too tight or clothing made of synthetic fabrics, which may trap heat and moisture and foster the development of germs.

Change Sanitary Products Regularly: To avoid bacterial development and lower your risk of infections, replace your sanitary items often *(at least every 4-6 hours)* if you use tampons or pads throughout your menstrual cycle.

Avoid Scented Items: Don't use scented pads, tampons, or other feminine care items. These goods may include irritants that might irritate the vagina or infect it by upsetting the normal bacterial balance.

Wipe from Front to Back: Always remember to wipe from front to back after peeing or having a bowel movement after using the toilet. This lessens the chance of urinary tract infections by preventing the spread of germs from the anal region to the urethra and vagina.

Maintain a Healthy Diet and Stay Hydrated: A balanced diet and enough water intake may assist to support overall vaginal health. Regular hydration aids in maintaining normal vaginal moisture and a balanced diet offers vital nutrients that support the body's defence systems.

It's best to get medical advice if you have any chronic itching, odd discharge, strong odour or pain in your intimate region in order to receive the right diagnosis and treatment.

Proper Cleansing Techniques

Maintaining excellent cleanliness and general vaginal health requires using the right washing methods for feminine intimate care. Here are some recommendations to remember:

Avoid using abrasive soaps, douches or scented items in the vaginal region by utilising gentle, unscented alternatives. They may irritate the body or infect it by upsetting the pH equilibrium naturally. Select gentle, fragrance-free soaps or cleansers made especially for intimate use.

Wash the external genital region carefully, paying particular attention to the vulva, or external vagina. Warm water and a light cleaner should be used to gently wash the area with your hand or a clean washcloth. Avoid using abrasive scrubbing since it might irritate the skin.

Rinsing properly is important to get rid of any cleanser residue left behind after cleaning. Irritation and pain might result from leftover soap or cleaner. Also douching or the use of a substance to flush water into the vagina, might upset the normal balance of vaginal flora.

The vagina is self-cleaning and typically has a stable pH level.

Following a thorough cleaning, gently wipe the area dry with a fresh towel. Roughly rubbing might irritate the skin; avoid doing so. Making sure the area is entirely dry is crucial since moisture might encourage the development of germs.

Use undergarments made of breathable, natural materials like cotton. Infection risk is decreased by these materials' ability to circulate air and aid in preventing moisture accumulation.

Avoid wearing clothing that is too tight; wearing clothing that is too tight, particularly trousers or synthetic fabrics, may trap heat and moisture, fostering the growth of germs and yeast. To encourage ventilation and lessen the chance of discomfort, choose loose-fitting clothes.

Immediately change out of sweaty or damp attire: A moist environment that encourages bacterial development may be produced by sitting for long periods of time in wet swimwear or sweaty clothing. To ensure cleanliness, change as soon as you can into dry clothing.

Most importantly maintaining good hygiene before and after sexual activity to practise safe sex. To keep it clean, wash your genital region with warm water and mild soap before and after sexual intercourse. In order to lower the risk of sexually transmitted infections (STIs), it's also crucial to utilise barrier techniques like condoms.

Choosing the Right Intimate Care Products

For adequate cleanliness and general vaginal health, choosing the appropriate personal care products is crucial. Here are some things to take into account while choosing intimate care products:

pH Balance: The vaginal pH is normally acidic and ranges from 3.8 to 4.5, which inhibits the development of dangerous bacteria. To preserve the vagina's natural acidity, look for intimate care products with a pH balance.

Mild Ingredients: Choose goods without abrasive chemicals, perfumes, colours, or sulphates. These have the potential to aggravate the sensitive skin around the vagina and throw off the vagina's normal balance.

Gentle Cleansers: Pick a vaginal cleanser that is made especially for the private parts of the body. Look for mild cleansers that are designed to remove dirt and grime without irritating or drying up the skin.

Options that are Natural and Organic: Some individuals like natural and organic items for intimate hygiene. These products could be kinder to sensitive skin since they might include less chemicals and synthetic components.

Allergies and Sensitivities: Carefully examine the ingredient list if you are aware of any known allergies or sensitivities to prevent any possible triggers. Prior to applying a new product to your intimate region, think about doing a patch test.

Douching is not advised since it might disturb the natural balance of the vagina and raise the risk of infections, so it's vital to keep that in mind. The vagina cleans itself and doesn't need to be doused.

Monthly Products: To maintain proper monthly hygiene, choose tampons, pads or menstrual cups that are constructed of permeable materials that are changed on a regular basis to avoid odour and bacterial development.

Seek Professional Advice: It is essential to visit a healthcare professional who can provide individualised advice and prescribe appropriate items if you have particular concerns or recurring difficulties with vaginal health.

Every individual has a unique physique, so what works for one person may not work for another. Pay attention to how your body reacts to various products, then modify as necessary.

THE IMPORTANCE OF PH BALANCE

Understanding pH and Its Impact

A solution's pH value indicates how basic or acidic it is. It calculates the amount of hydrogen ions (H+) present in a solution. The pH scale has a range of 0 to 14, with 7 being regarded as neutral. Acidic solutions have a pH below 7, whereas basic or alkaline solutions have a pH over 7.

Because of the logarithmic nature of the pH scale, each unit measures a tenfold change in acidity or basicity. For instance, a pH of 4 solution is ten times more acidic than a pH of 5 solution.

Numerous biological, chemical and environmental processes all depend heavily on pH.
Here are some of pH's main effects:

Biological Systems: The correct operation of biological systems depends on pH. The pH ranges within which an organism's enzymes and metabolic processes function best are particular. Variations from these pH ranges may have an impact on cellular function, protein structure and enzyme activity. For instance, to sustain typical physiological functions, the human body keeps the blood's pH at roughly 7.35-7.45, which is somewhat alkaline.

pH significantly affects aquatic habitats, especially in freshwater bodies of water. For life and reproduction, many aquatic creatures, including fish and invertebrates, have particular pH needs. These ecosystems' balances may be upset by acidic or basic water conditions, which can also affect the creatures that live there.

Water Quality: pH is a crucial factor in determining the quality of the water. To provide safe and appropriate drinking water, municipal water treatment facilities monitor pH levels and make adjustments as necessary. Furthermore, wastewater produced by industrial operations is often acidic or alkaline and has to be treated before it can be properly discharged back into the environment.

Chemical Reactions: The pace and result of many chemical reactions are influenced by pH. Some reactions are very pH-dependent, which means that they take place or develop in various ways depending on the pH level. For instance, the stability of pharmaceutical medications, the usefulness of certain cleaning chemicals or the performance of chemical reactions in industrial processes may all be impacted by the acidity or alkalinity of a solution.

Soil Fertility and Plant Growth: Plant development and soil fertility depend on the pH of the soil, which also affects nutrient availability. The pH of the soil may have an impact on the solubility of vital nutrients, and various plants have varying pH needs. Alkaline soils *(high pH)* may lead to nutritional imbalances, whereas acidic soils *(low pH)* might restrict the availability of certain nutrients. In order to provide the best growth conditions for crops, agriculture often modifies soil pH using techniques like liming or acidification.

Corrosion: The mechanisms of corrosion are influenced by pH. Acidic or alkaline conditions may hasten the corrosion of metals, resulting in the deterioration of materials, damage to infrastructure, and higher maintenance costs. Corrosion inhibitor use or maintaining proper pH levels in industrial processes may also aid in reducing these impacts.

Understanding pH is crucial for maintaining environmental balance, ensuring the appropriate operation of biological systems and improving industrial operations. Monitoring and regulating pH levels allows us to reduce negative impacts and foster ideal circumstances for a variety of applications.

Maintaining Optimal Vaginal pH

For general vaginal health and the prevention of many infections, maintaining an ideal vaginal pH is crucial. The vagina's usual pH range is 3.8 to 4.5, which is mildly acidic. ***Here are some pointers for maintaining a healthy vaginal pH:***

Practise good hygiene: Use mild, unscented soap and warm water to gently wash the external genital region to maintain excellent hygiene. As strong soaps, douches and feminine hygiene products might disturb the pH balance naturally, avoid using them.

Avoid using scented products: Keep your genital region free of scented soaps, bubble baths, powders and other items. These items have the ability to irritate the vagina and change its pH balance.

Wear breathable undergarments: Opt for undergarments made of natural fibres that breathe well, including cotton. Avoid wearing constrictive garments and synthetic fabrics, which may trap moisture and foster the growth of germs.

Avoid over-washing: Washing too much might upset the pH and microbial balance in the vaginal region. Avoid rough scrubbing and limit washing to once or twice daily for the exterior genital region.

Be mindful of sexual activity: Semen has an alkaline pH between 7 and 8, therefore use caution while engaging in sexual activity. The pH of the vagina might momentarily change during sexual activity, especially with a new partner or numerous partners. After sexual activity, urinating may help wash out any potentially dangerous germs and balance the pH.

Maintain a healthy diet: Eating a balanced diet full of fruits, vegetables, whole grains, and lean meats will help to maintain good vaginal health. According to certain research, consuming a lot of processed meals and refined sugars may be bad for your vaginal health.

Keep hydrated: Consuming enough water to maintain general hydration and may improve vaginal health.

Avoid unnecessary antibiotic use: Avoid using antibiotics until absolutely essential since they may upset the normal balance of germs in the vagina. Use antibiotics only when absolutely required and as directed by a medical practitioner.

Probiotics: Take into account adding probiotics to your daily regimen, either as a supplement or by ingesting foods that are high in good bacteria. A healthy balance of bacteria in the vagina may be maintained with the use of probiotics.

A healthcare provider should be seen if you have chronic vaginal pain, odd discharge, odour or other troubling symptoms in order to get an accurate diagnosis and the best course of action.

pH-Balanced Products and Their Benefits

Products with a pH balance are designed to match the natural pH of our skin or other bodily tissues. The pH scale, which spans from 0 to 14, is used to determine how acidic or alkaline a material is, with 7 being regarded as neutral. A pH value of 7 or above indicates alkalinity, whereas a pH value of 7 or below suggests acidity.

The following are a few advantages of utilising pH-balanced products:

Maintains the skin's natural barrier: The acid mantle, a thin layer that functions as a barrier against germs, pollution and other external irritants, is a natural defence mechanism for our skin. Using pH-balanced skincare products aids in preserving and supporting the acid mantle, a natural barrier with a slightly acidic pH level (about 5.5). pH balance is necessary for the skin to operate properly and maintain its health.

Non-irritating and kind to the skin: Products with a pH balance are designed to be kind to the skin, particularly for individuals who have sensitive or easily irritated skin. They assist in reducing the possibility of adverse skin responses, such as redness, dryness or stinging, which may happen when using products with high or low pH levels that disturb the skin's natural equilibrium.

Restores and maintains the skin hydration: pH-balanced cleansers and moisturisers may assist in controlling the skin's moisture levels. Restores and maintains the skin's hydration. These products are usually designed to be neither too moisturising nor underdrying, keeping the skin nourished without removing its natural oils. This is crucial for those with dry or dehydrated skin in particular.

Supports a healthy scalp: Shampoos and conditioners with a pH balance may support a healthy scalp. The pH of the scalp is naturally acidic, preventing microbial proliferation and preserving the general health of the hair and scalp. It is possible to avoid scalp problems like dandruff, itching and excessive oiliness by using pH-balanced hair care products.

Suitable for personal hygiene: The vaginal region's health is especially dependent on pH balance. The vagina's normal pH is somewhat acidic *(between 3.5 and 4.5)*, which aids in preventing the formation of dangerous germs and preserving a healthy vaginal flora. The vaginal pH can be maintained and imbalances that could cause infections or pain can be avoided by using pH-balanced intimate washes or other feminine care products.

It's very important to note that not every product needs a pH balance. For instance, certain skincare items, such as exfoliants or particular treatments, may purposefully have a variable pH for those purposes. However, maintaining a pH balance may be advantageous for general skin and body health when used for everyday usage or items that come into close contact with the skin or intimate regions.

MANAGING ODOUR AND DISCHARGE

Normal vs. Abnormal Odour and Discharge

Understanding what is normal and what can be an anomaly when it comes to feminine intimate care is crucial. *Here is a broad summary:*

Normal Odour: Every woman has her own distinct aroma and the vagina often has a moderate odour. The aroma is often characterised as somewhat musky or as being mildly pleasant. Throughout the menstrual cycle, this smell might alter, but it shouldn't be overpowering or unpleasant.

Normal Discharge: Vaginal discharge is a common occurrence that is essential to preserving vaginal health. By removing germs and dead cells, it keeps the vagina clean. Normal discharge may fluctuate in quality and amount during the menstrual cycle and is often clear or white.

Abnormal Odour: An abnormal odour coming from your vagina might be an indication of an infection if it is strong, nasty, fishy or otherwise unpleasant. A sexually transmitted infection *(STI)* or an illness like bacterial vaginosis may be indicated by a strong odour that is also accompanied by additional symptoms including itching, burning or discomfort. It's crucial in these situations to speak with a healthcare expert for a diagnosis and the best course of action.

Abnormal Discharge: Modifications in the colour, texture or volume of vaginal discharge may point to a problem. For instance, if the discharge thickens, clumps (like cottage cheese), becomes green, yellow or foams, it might be a sign of an illness like a yeast infection or a STI. It's also wise to get medical help if the discharge is accompanied by itchiness, burning, redness or discomfort.

Being aware of what is typical for you and paying attention to your body are both very important. It is essential to speak with a healthcare provider if you have any substantial changes in discharge or odour that worry you. If required, they can provide a precise diagnosis and suggest the best course of action.

Maintaining overall vaginal health requires controlling odour and discharge while providing feminine personal care.

Here are some pointers to assist you in controlling odour and discharge:

Good hygiene dictates that you gently wash your external genital region with warm water and a moderate, fragrance-free soap. The natural equilibrium of the vagina may be upset by using strong cleansers, douches or perfumed items, which can irritate the area.

Choose cotton undergarments to promote greater airflow and keep the vaginal region dry. Avoid wearing form-fitting pants or synthetic materials that might trap moisture and encourage the development of germs. No douching since it may throw off the pH balance of the vagina and encourage the development of dangerous germs. Douching is not necessary since the vagina cleans itself. The exterior genital region just needs to be washed.

Balanced diet that is high in fruits, vegetables and probiotics to promote vaginal health. Probiotics, which may be obtained as supplements or in yoghurt, can assist in maintaining a balanced population of bacteria in the vagina, also drinking enough water may encourage healthy vaginal discharge and aid in toxin removal.

Safe sexual behaviour may help lower the chance of acquiring vaginal odour and abnormal discharge as well as the transmission of sexually transmitted diseases *(STIs)*.

Use scented goods sparingly; fragrances, such as those found in scented tampons, pads and toilet paper, may irritate the delicate vaginal region. Instead, use items that are odourless or fragrance-free. If you use tampons or pads during your period, do so to avoid bacteria growth and odour. If possible, use pads or tampons made of natural materials.

Avoid wearing tight clothes because it may trap heat and moisture in the vaginal region, which can encourage the development of germs. Whenever possible, choose comfortable, loose-fitting clothes.

Most especially, It's essential to speak with a healthcare provider if you detect any persistent or odd changes in your vaginal odour or discharge. They can provide the proper therapy or guidance while also assisting in identifying any underlying problems.

Keep in mind that a faint odour and discharge, which might change during your menstrual cycle, are typical for the vagina. However, it's critical to get medical assistance if you suffer any of the following symptoms: a strong, disagreeable odour; itching; burning; or odd changes in discharge. These symptoms might be indicators of an infection or other underlying problem.

Natural Remedies and Lifestyle Changes

Certainly! Consider the following additional all-natural cures and lifestyle modifications while practising feminine intimate care:

Balanced diet: A healthy diet helps improve vaginal health in general. Include a range of fresh produce in your meals, along with whole grains, lean meats and healthy fats. This may strengthen your immune system and keep your vaginal health at its best.

Keep moving: Regular exercise encourages good blood circulation, which is advantageous for the vaginal region. Improve your general blood flow by doing exercises like walking, running, swimming, or yoga to maintain healthy vaginal function.

Avoid smoking and drinking too much alcohol: These behaviours might disturb the normal balance of bacteria in the vagina and raise the risk of infections. To preserve vaginal health, give up smoking and consume alcohol sparingly or not at all.

Consider using water-based lubricants if you have vaginal dryness during sexual activity to increase comfort. Avoid using silicone- or petroleum-based lubricants, since these may disrupt the vagina's normal pH balance.

Practise safe and gentle hair removal: Use mild and safe hair removal techniques if you decide to wax your pubic area to reduce discomfort and ingrown hairs. Strong hair removal lotions or forceful shaving methods may not be as effective as trimming, using a clean blade or professional waxing.

Maintain a healthy weight: Being overweight increases the likelihood of perspiration and moisture accumulation, which may lead to bacterial development and illnesses. By eating a balanced diet and getting regular exercise, work towards a healthy weight range.

Practise good bathroom habits: Maintain proper bathroom habits by constantly wiping from front to back while using the toilet to stop germs from spreading from the anal region to the vagina. This little action may assist in lowering the risk of vaginal problems and UTIs.

Avoid extended moisture: Immediately change out of damp or sweaty clothing after engaging in activities like swimming or working out. Long-term wetness in the vaginal region may foster the development of germs and promote infections.

Sleep hygiene: Prioritise getting a good night's sleep to support your overall health, which includes your vaginal health. For your immune system to be strengthened and to assist control hormonal balance, aim for seven to eight hours of good sleep each night.

Regular health check-ups: Gynaecological screenings and check-ups should be scheduled on a regular basis with your healthcare practitioner. Regular examinations may guarantee general vaginal health by assisting in the early detection of any possible problems.

Always pay attention to your body's signals and seek medical attention if you have any worries or persistent symptoms. Finding the techniques and treatments that are most effective for you is essential since every person is different.

NURTURING INTIMATE WELLNESS

Maintaining Vaginal Health

To continue preserving vaginal health, consider the following advice:

Use the right wiping technique by always wiping from front to back on the toilet after urinating or removing your waste. The incidence of urinary tract infections *(UTIs)* and other infections is decreased because of this because it helps stop the movement of germs from the anal region to the vagina. Exercise regularly to maintain good blood flow to the pelvic area and to boost general circulation. The immune system is strengthened as well and this may assist maintain the health of the vagina.

Avoid sitting in damp clothing for a lengthy amount of time. This may increase bacterial development by creating a moist atmosphere. To keep the vaginal region dry and avoid dangerous infections, immediately remove any moist clothes. DO NOT misuse antibiotics, they may upset the normal balance of bacteria in the vagina even if they are required for treating bacterial infections. With the goal of reducing the usage of antibiotics, wherever feasible, talk to your doctor about alternative therapies or preventative measures.

Know your options when it comes to birth control: Some options, such spermicides or diaphragms, may cause discomfort or have an impact on the pH of the vagina. Discuss alternative methods with your healthcare professional if you feel any pain or changes in the health of your vagina after using a certain type of contraception.

Smoking raises your chance of getting vaginal infections among other health problems. The vaginal microbiota may be impacted by excessive alcohol intake, which also makes infections more likely to occur. It is possible to improve vaginal health by leading a healthy lifestyle that includes quitting smoking and drinking in moderation.

It's crucial to be careful when using lubricants, vaginal washes or intimate sprays. Choose items formulated for vaginal pH and sensitive skin. Before utilising new items, speak with a medical practitioner if you have any worries or allergies.

Preventing Infections: Yeast, Bacterial Vaginosis, and UTIs

Here are some extra precautions and ideas for avoiding certain infections:

Yeast Infections:

Avoid wearing clothes that fit tightly because it may trap heat and moisture, which is the perfect habitat for yeast to develop. This goes double for synthetic fabrics.

As soon as you can, change out of wet or damp clothing, such as swimsuits or sweaty gym attire. Wash your pants with a moderate, unscented laundry detergent instead of fabric softener or dryer sheets, which may contain irritants. Consider avoiding or lowering your consumption of foods rich in yeast or sugar if you regularly have yeast infections since they may promote overgrowth. Bread, beer, wine and sweet treats may be among them.

BV, or Bacterial Vaginosis:

Douching should be avoided since it might alter the normal balance of bacteria in the vagina and raise the risk of BV. When having a sexual encounter, use condoms since BV is linked to changing or having several partners.

Make sure the soaps or washes you use for vaginal hygiene are pH-balanced and particularly made for the vaginal region.

UTIs _(urinary tract infections)_:

Drink a lot of water throughout the day to stay hydrated. This aids in clearing germs from the urinary system. Regularly and thoroughly empty your bladder since holding onto pee for a long time might encourage the growth of germs.

Urinate and drink a full glass of water after sexual activity to help flush out any germs that may have entered the urethra.

Avoid applying potentially irritating personal care items to the genital region, such as abrasive soaps or feminine sprays.

If you often have UTIs, you may want to discuss taking a low-dose antibiotic or other preventative measures with your healthcare physician. Though taking these precautions may dramatically lower your chance of infection, it's still vital to consult a doctor if you get symptoms or have repeated illnesses. Your healthcare professional can provide an accurate diagnosis and suggest suitable treatments that are catered to your unique circumstances.

Addressing Common Vaginal Issues

Women often have vaginal problems, which may range in severity from minor annoyance to more severe infections. The best course of action is to speak with a healthcare professional if your symptoms are severe or chronic in order to get an accurate diagnosis and treatment plan.

Insufficient arousal during sexual activity, hormonal changes, certain drugs or vaginal dryness may all cause this condition. Using water-based lubricants during sexual activity may help ease pain. For long-term comfort, over-the-counter vaginal moisturisers are another option. For additional assessment, speak with a healthcare professional if dryness is uncomfortable and persistent.

Vaginal odour: The vagina often has a moderate, musky odour. A strong, disagreeable smell, however, can be a sign of an illness like bacterial vaginosis or a sexually transmitted infection (STI). It's crucial to see a healthcare professional for an assessment and the proper course of action if you experience a persistent or offensive odour.

Vaginal irritation: A number of conditions, including yeast infections, bacterial vaginosis, allergies or irritants such soaps or laundry detergents, may result in vaginal itching. Use mild, fragrance-free cleansers instead of scented ones on your genital region to avoid using scented products. It is advised to seek medical assistance if itching is persistent or accompanied by an unusual discharge.

Vaginal discharge: Regular vaginal discharge may vary in consistency during the menstrual cycle and is normally clear or milky in colour. However, an infection may be indicated by changes in colour, consistency, odour or increased discharge. Consult a healthcare professional if you have an unusual or troublesome discharge for a precise diagnosis and the best course of action.

Vaginal infections: Yeast infections and bacterial vaginosis are common vaginal infections. Itching, a thick white discharge, and redness are the usual symptoms of yeast infections. Uncomplicated yeast infections may be treated with over-the-counter antifungal medications, but it's best to speak with a doctor if you're uncertain or your symptoms don't go away. A thin, greyish-white discharge with a fishy odour is often the first sign of bacterial vaginosis. For diagnosis and treatment of bacterial vaginosis, it's crucial to speak with a healthcare professional as antibiotics are often given.

Urinary tract infections *(UTIs)*: When bacteria enter the urethra, they go up into the bladder, where they cause UTIs. Frequent urination, a strong need to pee, a burning feeling when urinating, and cloudy or bloody urine are all symptoms. Drink lots of water, urinate before and after sexual activity, and practise basic hygiene habits to help avoid UTIs. It's crucial to see a doctor if you think you have a UTI since antibiotics are usually required for diagnosis and treatment.

Recurring yeast infections *(recurrent yeast infections, or VVC)*: Itching, redness, swelling, and a thick, white discharge are symptoms of VVC, sometimes referred to as recurrent yeast infections. For minor infections, over-the-counter antifungal creams or suppositories may be used, but if symptoms persist or come back repeatedly, it's crucial to see a doctor for a correct diagnosis and course of treatment since there may be underlying conditions causing the recurring infections.

Sexually transmitted infections *(STIs)*: This may result in vaginal symptoms including abnormal discharge, itching, burning or blisters. STIs include chlamydia, gonorrhoea, trichomoniasis and herpes. It's critical to visit a healthcare professional for testing, diagnosis and proper treatment if you think you may have a STI or have participated in unsafe sexual behaviour. STI risk may be decreased by engaging in safe sex and utilising barrier techniques like condoms.

PID, also known as **Pelvic Inflammatory Disease**, is an infection of the reproductive organs that is often brought on by untreated STIs. Pelvic discomfort, unusual vaginal discharge, uncomfortable sex and fever are possible symptoms. It's crucial to get quick medical help if you have these symptoms since PID may cause major problems if neglected.

Genital Irritation and Allergies: Certain items, such as scented soaps, detergents or synthetic pants, may occasionally induce genital discomfort or allergic responses. Choosing mild, fragrance-free products and avoiding irritants may help treat symptoms.

Vaginal Health at Different Stages of Life

Women's general well being includes their vaginal health throughout their lifetimes. At various periods of life, there might be a wide range of vaginal health requirements and difficulties.

The following is a summary of the many phases of vaginal health considerations:

Puberty and Adolescence: Hormonal changes during puberty cause the commencement of menstruation and the development of secondary sexual traits. Young females should be taught good hygiene habits such as regular bathing, wearing clean pants and often changing period products. It's also advised to stay away from douching, perfumed items and tight clothes since these things might irritate the vaginal flora and throw off its normal balance.

Reproductive Years: Menstruation, sexual activity and delivery are all possible throughout the reproductive years for women. It's crucial to practise safe sex, use the proper sanitary products, and maintain excellent menstrual hygiene. The importance of routine cervical cancer and STI screening cannot be overstated. Additionally, it's important to inform your medical team if you have any odd vaginal discharge, pain or menstrual cycle abnormalities.

Pregnancy: Hormonal changes that occur during pregnancy might have an impact on vaginal health. Vaginal discharge may become more frequent due to hormonal changes and increased blood flow to the pelvic area. It's critical to practise proper hygiene and put on permeable pants. To prevent irritation, stay away from douching and use gentle, fragrance-free products. Women who are expecting should talk to their doctors about any worries they have, particularly if they relate to infections or changes in vaginal discharge.

Menopause and Perimenopause: As women approach menopause and perimenopause, hormonal changes result in a drop in oestrogen levels, which causes vaginal dryness, vaginal atrophy, and pH changes in the vaginal fluid. These modifications may cause pain, itchiness and a higher chance of urinary tract infections (UTIs). Dryness may be reduced by regular sexual activity or by using lubricants or moisturisers. Some women may also choose hormone replacement treatment (HRT), however this should be addressed with a healthcare professional.

Postmenopause: Due to the increased likelihood of vaginal atrophy and its accompanying symptoms after menopause, preserving vaginal health becomes even more crucial. The vaginal tissues may be kept healthy by engaging in regular sexual activity or by using lubricants and moisturisers in the vagina. Additionally, regular cervical and vaginal screenings as well as gynaecological checks should continue.

Postpartum: The body undergoes a healing phase after delivery. During this period, vaginal discomfort, edema and discharge are frequent occurrences. Infections may be avoided by practising good hygiene, which includes taking frequent baths and keeping the perineal region clean. To enable the body to repair correctly after postpartum bleeding, sanitary pads are advised rather than tampons.

Elderly Age: As we get older, hormonal changes, decreased oestrogen levels and underlying medical issues may all have an impact on our vaginal health. Inconvenience during sexual activity and a higher risk of UTIs may result from vaginal shrinkage and dryness. Vaginal health at this stage may be managed by regular sexual activity, the use of lubricants and moisturisers and maintaining general health. Additionally, it's crucial to discuss any worries with a healthcare professional since they may advise on available treatments and preventative actions.

Chronic Health Conditions: Women with long-term health issues, such diabetes or autoimmune diseases, may be more susceptible to vaginal infections and pain. For the purpose of preserving vaginal health, the underlying problem must be treated well. In order to monitor and handle any particular issues with vaginal health in the context of chronic diseases, it's crucial to engage closely with healthcare specialists.

Psychiatric and emotional health:
At every stage of life, psychological and emotional wellness are equally important for vaginal health. Hormone levels and vaginal health may be affected by stress, anxiety and certain drugs. Vaginal health may be improved by using stress reduction strategies, leading a healthy lifestyle and taking care of any mental health issues.

SEXUAL WELLNESS AND INTIMACY

Sexual Health Education

The provision of accurate and age-appropriate information regarding sexual and reproductive health is a key component of comprehensive health education. It covers a broad variety of subjects, including but not limited to:

Anatomy and Physiology: Instruction on the structures and processes that make up the male and female reproductive systems.

Puberty: Menstruation, growth spurts and hormone changes are just a few of the physical and psychological changes that happen throughout puberty.

Reproduction: Understanding the fundamentals of human reproduction, including conception, pregnancy and delivery.

Contraception: Understanding the many kinds of contraceptive techniques, their efficacy and the proper way to use them.

Sexual Transmitted Infections (STIs): Information about common sexually transmitted infections (STIs), their means of transmission, methods of prevention and the value of routine testing.

Consent: Establishing limits, learning what constitutes healthy and consenting sexual behaviour, and receiving education about the significance of permission in sexual relationships are all parts of the concept of consent.

Healthy Relationships: Promote knowledge of good relationships, communication abilities, respect and the significance of identifying and resolving problems including coercion, manipulation and abuse.

Gender and Sexual Orientation: Encouragement of acceptance, understanding and tolerance for all gender identities and sexual orientations.

Self-esteem and Body Image: Addressing the cultural pressures placed on individuals' perceptions of their bodies and fostering healthy self-esteem and body positivity.

Responsible Decision-Making: Encourage critical thought and decision-making abilities when it comes to sexual behaviour, relationships and personal beliefs.

Online Safety: Internet, social media and other digital platforms should be used responsibly and with awareness of the possible threats, according to online safety.

More other components of teaching on sexual health:

Communication Skills: Teaching good communication techniques, such as assertiveness, bargaining and active listening, to improve communication in partnerships and sexual experiences.

Pleasure and Intimacy: Recognising and appreciating the value of pleasure, closeness and emotional health in sexual interactions.

Emotional Aspects of Sexuality: Discussing the emotional sides of sexuality, such as feelings of attraction and love as well as how to control your feelings during a sexual encounter.

Responsible Sexual Behaviour: Promoting responsible sexual behaviour, emphasising the value of open communication, trust and respect between couples.

Pregnancy Choices: Informing people about their alternatives during pregnancy, such as parenting, adoption and abortion and offering them nonjudgmental support.

Prevention of Sexual Violence: Sexual violence may be prevented by addressing the problem, fostering consent understanding and healthy relationships and offering options for reporting and getting treatment.

Cultural and Religious Considerations: Providing accurate and comprehensive information while acknowledging and honouring various cultural and religious views on sexuality.

Access to Sexual Health Care: Informing people about the accessibility of sexual healthcare services, such as STI testing, contraception and reproductive health services and removing access-related obstacles.

Media Literacy: The ability to assess and analyse sexuality-related media messages, such as unrealistic body standards, pornography and advertising, requires the development of critical thinking abilities.

Rights and Advocacy: Promoting advocacy for sexual and reproductive health concerns while educating about sexual rights, such as the right to a thorough sexuality education, access to healthcare and freedom from discrimination.

Comprehensive, research-based and age-appropriate sexual health education should be offered. As well as respecting personal values and beliefs, it should take into account cultural sensitivity. People who receive effective sexual health education have the information, abilities and attitudes needed to make wise choices, support good relationships and maintain their sexual health and wellbeing throughout the course of their life.

Communicating with Partners about Intimate Care

Open and honest communication is essential when it comes to discussing personal care with your spouse. *Here are some suggestions for handling this delicate subject:*

Pick the ideal moment and location: Find a quiet, secluded location where you and your spouse may speak without interruption. Don't talk about private problems in front of others or while you or your partner are anxious or preoccupied.

Create a Non-Judgmental Environment: Establish a secure and accepting atmosphere by making sure your spouse feels secure and welcomed while talking about intimate care. Don't be critical or judgmental and make it clear that you're talking to them about improving your relationship because you care about their well-being.

Making "I" statements To avoid seeming accusatory or aggressive, frame your worries or objectives using "I" phrases. Say, "I've been considering our intimate care routine and I feel like we could explore some new options together," as an example. How do you feel?

Be Explicit and Precise: Express your ideas, worries or aspirations about intimate care in clear terms. This clarifies your viewpoint for your spouse and invites their contribution to the dialogue. If necessary, provide concrete instances; nevertheless, keep your partner's sentiments in mind.

Listen Actively: Actively listen to your partner's ideas, emotions and worries about intimate care. Allow them the time and space to do so. Focus on what they are saying, be sure you look them in the eye and respond in a way that is encouraging and sympathetic. Don't interrupt or make snap judgements.

Respect Personal Space: Everyone has their own comfort zones and limits when it comes to intimate care. Observe the preferences and restrictions of your spouse. Establish mutual consent and limits by talking about what you both find comfortable.

Together, look for solutions: Assume that the dialogue is a team effort. Together, come up with ideas and solutions to enhance your intimate care regimen. Think about looking into new possibilities, experimenting with other tools or methods or even consulting a professional if required.

Continually communicate with your spouse. Since intimate care is a continuous activity, make it a point to do so. Inquire about their feelings and any modifications or improvements they would want to see. Encourage them to provide comments and be open to their ideas.

Normalise the conversation by pointing out that intimate care is a normal and natural component of preserving general health and wellbeing. Recognising that it's a subject worth addressing honestly and without shame can help normalise the discourse. Stressing that you are on the same team, encourage your spouse to express their ideas and worries.

Educate one another: Use this chance to educate one another if you or your spouse are unaware of or misinformed about intimate care procedures. To get correct information, read articles from reputable sources, talk to medical experts or do research. Sharing this procedure may promote cohesion and shared accountability.

Be Attentive to Emotions: Talking about intimate care may sometimes cause delicate feelings, anxieties, or memories of the past. Be aware of this and approach the discussion with compassion and sensitivity. Verify your partner's emotions and tell them that you are there to help them while they face any difficulties.

Focus on pleasure and intimacy: Highlight the link between intimate care and pleasure, closeness and overall relationship satisfaction rather than just viewing intimate care from a practical or sanitary standpoint. Talk about strategies to make your personal encounters more sensual and emotional.

Experiment and be Open-minded: Try new things and have an open mind since everyone has different intimate hygiene practices. Encourage experimentation and an open mind while attempting new strategies, items, or methods. This may keep the discussion lively, engaging and receptive to one another's changing demands.

Discuss the topic again if necessary. Age, health and changes in lifestyle are just a few examples of the many reasons that might cause intimate care preferences and requirements to vary over time. To make sure that your personal care routines continue to satisfy both your needs and desires, make it a practice to revisit the topic from time to time. Be willing to modify and adapt as required.

Celebrate Progress and Successes: Recognise and applaud any improvements or advancements you and your partner achieve in your intimate care routines. Recognise the efforts made by both spouses and show your gratitude for how you are promoting each other's wellbeing.

Do note that good communication about intimate care requires continual discussion, mutual respect and awareness of one another's limits. Your personal connection may be strengthened and a stronger, more rewarding relationship can be fostered by placing a high priority on open communication, mutual support and shared responsibility.

Safe Sex Practices and Protection: Postpartum Care and Recovery

It's crucial to look after your body and give it time to recuperate after giving birth. Safe sex practices and protection should be taken into consideration when it comes to postpartum treatment and recovery. *Following are some pointers to bear in mind:*

Delay till you're prepared: Before starting up again, give yourself adequate time to recover physically and emotionally. In order to guarantee appropriate healing, healthcare professionals often advise waiting at least six weeks following a vaginal birth or until the postpartum check-up.

Talk to your partner about how you feel and any worries you have about starting up your sexual activity again. To make sure that both spouses are on the same page throughout this period, open communication is essential.

Consider using contraception if you don't immediately aim to become pregnant in order to avoid an unplanned pregnancy. Discuss your alternatives with your healthcare professional, taking into account aspects including breastfeeding, general health and personal preferences.

Barrier techniques: Barrier techniques, such as condoms and dental dams, may give extra layers of contraception while protecting against STIs. STI transmission may be decreased by routinely and appropriately using condoms during sexual activity.

Lubrication: Vaginal dryness may sometimes be brought on by nursing and hormonal changes after childbirth. To improve comfort and lessen any pain or discomfort during sexual activity, think about using a water-based lubricant.

Exercises for the Pelvic floor: Performing pelvic floor exercises, sometimes referred to as "Kegels," may assist to strengthen the pelvic muscles, enhance bladder control and hasten recuperation. Better sexual health and pleasure may be attributed to strong pelvic floor muscles.

Be kind and patient; understand that pregnancy and motherhood have caused enormous changes to your body. When engaging in sexual activity, go gently, pay attention to your body and put your comfort and wellbeing first.

Seek Professional help if needed: If you feel ongoing pain, discomfort or other problems during or during sexual activity, don't hesitate to speak with your healthcare physician. In order to address any issues, they may provide direction, support and sometimes even treatment alternatives.

Get tested for sexually transmitted infections (STIs) if you or your partner have had sexual contact with anybody during the postpartum period. Regular testing helps to safeguard your partner's health as well as your own.

Breastfeeding and Contraception: It's crucial to keep in mind that certain hormonal contraceptive techniques might influence a nursing mother's milk supply. Ask your doctor about methods of contraception that you may take while still nursing.

Contraceptive Choices: Your options for contraception may include birth control pills, hormonal patches, intrauterine devices (IUDs), contraceptive implants or injectables, depending on your preferences and medical history. The ideal decision for you may be determined with the aid of your healthcare practitioner.

Emotional preparedness: It's important to deal with any emotional shifts or worries that may occur throughout the postpartum time. It's crucial to talk with your spouse and ask for help if necessary since being a parent may result in a range of feelings. Relationship pleasure and sexual intimacy are both influenced by emotional health.

Breast or nipple sensitivity: You may need to modify your sexual activities if you are suffering breast or nipple sensitivity as a result of nursing. To alleviate pain, try alternate positions or look into non-breast-focused sexual activities.

Postpartum Bleeding: After giving birth, you may continue to suffer postpartum bleeding or discharge *(lochia)* for the first several weeks. To prevent any mess or pain, it's crucial to wear the right protection, such as pads, during sexual activity

Keep up with postpartum changes: Become familiar with the physical changes that take place at this time, such as changes in breast size and sensitivity, perineal pain and vaginal dryness. Being prepared for these changes might make it easier for you to deal with them.

Every person's postpartum experience is different, so it's important to prioritise self-care, pay attention to your body and be honest with your spouse. The greatest source for individualised information and assistance based on your unique requirements and circumstances is your healthcare practitioner.

Understanding the Changes After Pregnancy

For a woman's body, pregnancy is an extraordinary and changing event. Numerous physiological, hormonal and emotional changes are brought about, all of which are necessary for the baby's healthy growth and development. Women go through a postpartum period after pregnancy during which their bodies progressively recuperate and acclimatise to the new stage of parenting.

Following pregnancy, the following changes are frequent:

Weight changes: Women put on weight throughout pregnancy to support the growing baby. Due to the baby, placenta and amniotic fluid being expelled after delivery, they often lose weight right after. However, it's common to gain back some weight after giving birth, especially in the form of excess body fat. The amount of time it takes to lose the remaining weight varies from woman to woman.

Breast changes: The breasts change significantly throughout pregnancy in order to prepare for lactation. The breasts begin producing milk after delivery, which may make them engorged, bigger and more sensitive. The breasts progressively recover to their pre-pregnancy size if nursing continues, however they may not be precisely the same as before if a woman decides not to breastfeed.

Hormonal changes: Hormone levels undergo significant change throughout pregnancy and they continue to change after delivery. Progesterone and oestrogen levels, which rise throughout pregnancy, sharply decline after delivery. In some women, these hormonal changes might cause mood swings, the postpartum blues or even postpartum depression.

Abdominal changes: The muscles and skin of the abdomen extend during pregnancy to make room for the developing foetus. Following birth, the uterus shrinks and eventually regains its pre-pregnancy size. Even so, it can take weeks or even months for the skin to tighten and the abdominal muscles to fully recover. Diastasis recti, when the abdominal muscles separate, may occur in certain women and has to be treated with particular exercises.

Changes to the pelvic floor: During pregnancy and delivery, the pelvic floor muscles, which support the bladder, uterus, and intestines, are put under a lot of strain. Weakening of the pelvic floor muscles as a consequence of this may cause problems like pelvic organ prolapse or urine incontinence. Exercises for the pelvic floor, sometimes referred to as Kegel exercises, may assist to strengthen these muscles.

Hair and Skin changes: Hormonal changes during pregnancy may result in changes to the hair and skin. Some women postpartum report having thicker, glossier hair, while others could suffer greater hair losing. Similar modifications may occur to the skin, such flare-ups of acne or the emergence of dark patches. Usually only transitory, these alterations eventually disappear.

Emotional adjustment: A variety of feelings, from delight and excitement to fear and mood swings, may be experienced throughout pregnancy and delivery. Women who just gave birth may go through the "baby blues," which include mood fluctuations, impatience and emotional instability. It's crucial to seek medical attention if these feelings intensify or continue since it may be a sign of postpartum depression.

Vaginal alterations: During pregnancy and delivery, the vaginal region may experience a variety of changes. Increased vaginal discharge, dryness or sensitivity may result from the increased blood flow and hormonal changes. The vagina may feel strained or painful after delivery. The vaginal tissues and muscles usually restore their tone over time, although it might take some time. Kegel exercises may aid in pelvic floor muscle strengthening and vaginal healing.

Joint and ligament slackness: To prepare for delivery, the body produces hormones throughout pregnancy that relax the ligaments and joints. The extra weight of pregnancy combined with this looseness might strain the joints. Some women may have joint stiffness or instability during this time as the ligaments and joints require some time to restore to their pre-pregnancy form.

Postpartum bleeding: After giving birth, women endure postpartum bleeding, sometimes referred to as lochia. This bleeding might linger for a few weeks and is comparable to a heavy menstrual cycle. The bleeding may start out bright red and gradually change to a milder shade. Use the proper sanitary products and if you have questions about heavy bleeding or other strange symptoms, go to a doctor.

Changes in sleep patterns: Because of the baby's feeding schedule and the difficulties of caring for a newborn, sleep interruptions are frequent after delivery. With many nighttime awakenings, new moms usually have fragmented sleep. Fatigue and drowsiness throughout the day may result from this. These changes may be managed by establishing a sleep schedule and asking for assistance from a spouse or family members.

Maternal instincts and emotional bonding: After giving birth, many women feel a strong sense of love and affection for their unborn child. This feeling is referred to as bonding. Many mothers grow confidence in their capacity to care for their kid as their maternal instincts mature. Bonding occasions may differ from person to person, however, and some mothers may need some time to acclimatise and forge a solid emotional tie with their offspring.

Nurturing Physical and Emotional Recovery

A crucial component of total wellbeing and healing is nurturing physical and emotional recovery. Taking intentional measures to promote your recovery may dramatically speed up the healing process, regardless of whether you're recuperating from a physical injury, sickness or a difficult emotional period.

Here are some ideas for promoting both physical and psychological recovery:

Rest and relaxation: Give yourself plenty of time to recharge. Pay attention to your body's needs and give enough rest and relaxation first priority. Allowing yourself to take pauses can help you avoid pushing yourself too hard too quickly.

Nutrition and Hydration: Maintain a healthy, balanced diet to aid in your physical recuperation. Drink plenty of water. Make sure you're receiving the nutrition you need and keeping hydrated. If necessary, get advice from a nutritionist or healthcare provider.

Exercise gently: Take part in activities that are mild and supportive of your recuperation. To learn what workouts are suitable for you and that are safe, speak with your healthcare physician. Exercise may increase blood flow, movement and endorphin production, all of which can boost mental wellbeing.

Seek Professional Advice: If you're experiencing emotional difficulties, you may want to think about getting professional advice. A therapist, counsellor or psychologist may provide helpful assistance, direction and coping mechanisms to help you successfully navigate your emotional recovery.

Support System: Surround yourself with a network of loved ones, close friends, or support organisations. Having understanding and sympathetic friends and family members may be consoling and emotionally supportive throughout the healing process.

Self-Care Activities: Take part in self-care exercises that encourage unwinding, stress relief and emotional wellbeing. This might include routines like journaling, mindfulness training, deep breathing exercises, meditation or participating in enjoyable activities.

Create Realistic Expectations: Be honest with yourself about your healing process and try not to put too much pressure on it. Recognise that recovery takes time and that setbacks might happen. Instead of concentrating on perfection, focus on progress and acknowledge minor wins along the way.

Practise Positive Thinking: Develop a positive mentality by engaging in positive thinking. Confront negative beliefs and swap them out with stronger, more empowered ones. Surround yourself with uplifting reading, inspiring phrases and affirmations.

Do Things That Make You Happy: Do things that make you happy, whether they include being in nature, indulging in hobbies you like, listening to music, reading or making art. These pursuits may provide satisfaction, diversion and emotional well-being.

Self-Compassion and Patience: Throughout your recuperation, practise self-compassion and patience. Recognise that recovery takes time and that obstacles are a normal part of the path. Be kind to yourself and give yourself frequent self-care.

Practise Relaxation and Mindfulness Techniques: Practise deep breathing, gradual muscular relaxation, mindfulness meditation or other relaxation methods. These techniques may aid in stress reduction, emotional wellness and self-awareness enhancement.

Engage in creative expression via writing, drawing, playing an instrument, dancing or other activities. Creative expression may be therapeutic, aid in the processing of emotions and provide happiness and a feeling of fulfilment.

Practise Gratitude: Make a habit of thinking about the things you have to be thankful for. By focusing on the good parts of your life, this practice may help you feel more satisfied and resilient.

Seek Social Support: Through support groups or online forums, find others who have gone through comparable struggles. Sharing your struggles, worries and successes with like-minded people may be reassuring and insightful.

Maintain limits: It's essential to establish limits throughout your rehabilitation in order to safeguard your physical and mental wellbeing. Saying no to obligations or activities that can overwhelm you or impede your development will help. Set your requirements in order of importance and let people know what they are.

Develop Positive Relationships: Surround yourself with positive, encouraging individuals. Spend time with loved ones who make your life better, creating a setting that is soothing and emotionally healthy.

Practise Self-Compassion: Recognise that rehabilitation requires time and effort and treat yourself with kindness and gentleness. You should treat yourself with the same compassion and care that you would provide to a loved one going through a similar situation.

Laugh therapy should be used since laughter has potent therapeutic effects. Take part in amusing activities, spend time with humorous people or watch comedy programmes. Laughter may elevate mood, lower stress levels and enhance general wellbeing.

Investigate Holistic Therapies: Take into account alternative treatments like acupuncture, massage, yoga or aromatherapy. These techniques may ease physical tension, encourage relaxation and aid in mental recovery.

Celebrate Success: Throughout your recovery path, be sure to recognise and honour your successes. Take some time to reflect on your progress and give yourself a reward, whether it's a little victory or a major milestone.

Everybody's rehabilitation is different, so it's important to tailor these recommendations to your own needs and preferences. On your journey to physical and mental rehabilitation, exercise patience, perseverance and an open mind to learning what works best for you.

Caring for the Pelvic Floor

Both men and women should take good care of their pelvic floors because they support the pelvic organs, maintain bowel and bladder control, and promote sexual function. Following are some crucial elements of pelvic floor care:

Exercise: Regular Kegel exercises, commonly known as pelvic floor exercises, may help the pelvic floor muscles become stronger. To do Kegels, locate the muscles that are utilised to interrupt the midstream flow of pee and squeeze them for a brief period of time before letting go. Aim for three daily sessions of 10 repetitions. Walking and other low-impact exercises may assist maintain general pelvic floor health on a regular basis.

Maintain a healthy weight since being overweight may strain the pelvic floor and cause weakness or dysfunction. Such problems may be avoided by maintaining a healthy weight with a balanced diet and frequent exercise.

Good bowel habits: Constipation may weaken the pelvic floor muscles if you strain to go. Make sure your food is high in fibre, drink plenty of water and schedule frequent bowel movements if you want to maintain good bowel habits. Refrain from putting off the impulse to go to the toilet.

Methods to utilise while lifting heavy goods: To prevent placing too much stress on the pelvic floor, it is vital to adopt the right methods when lifting large objects. Lift using your legs rather than your back or pelvic region, keeping your back straight. Injuries to the pelvic floor are less likely as a result.

Avoid strenuous workouts with high impact: Activities like sprinting and leaping may strain the pelvic floor. Consider low-impact workouts as alternatives if you have a weak pelvic floor or are having pelvic floor dysfunction, such as swimming or cycling.

Maintain proper posture; poor posture may put undue strain on the muscles of the pelvic floor. To reduce pelvic floor tension, concentrate on keeping your posture erect when sitting and standing.

Seek therapy for pelvic floor problems: It's critical to speak with a healthcare provider who specialises in treating pelvic floor disorders if you are exhibiting symptoms like urine incontinence, pelvic discomfort or prolapsed pelvic organs. They can identify the problem and suggest the best course of action, which may include pelvic floor physical therapy, medication or surgical procedures.

Practice Relaxation techniques: Use relaxation strategies to reduce stress and tension, which may lead to pelvic floor problems. Learning and using relaxation methods like yoga, deep breathing exercises and mindfulness helps ease pelvic floor muscle tension and enhance general calm.

Be Mindful of chronic constipation: Keep in mind that persistent constipation may put pressure on the pelvic floor and result in problems like pelvic organ prolapse. Maintain a diet rich in fibre, drink plenty of water and, if necessary, use light stool softeners or fibre supplements to avoid constipation. Consult a doctor if constipation doesn't go away.

Control persistent coughing: The muscles in the pelvic floor might get sore from repeated, powerful coughing. Seek proper medical therapy if you have a persistent cough, such as one brought on by asthma or a respiratory illness, to lessen the effect it has on your pelvic floor.

Avoid sitting for extended periods of time: Prolonged sitting might cause pelvic floor problems. Try to take frequent pauses to stand, stretch and move about if your work demands a lot of sitting. Use pillows or seats that are ergonomically built to reduce strain on the pelvic floor.

Get ready for delivery: The pelvic floor may experience tremendous tension throughout pregnancy and childbirth. It is advantageous to do pregnancy activities that concentrate on the pelvic floor, including prenatal yoga or Pilates, with the assistance of a trained teacher. Restart pelvic floor exercises gradually after giving birth and get medical advice if you have any postpartum pelvic floor problems.

Avoid lifting heavy objects when pregnant since doing so puts more strain on the pelvic floor. In order to avoid placing undue pressure on the pelvic floor muscles, avoid heavy lifting and ask for help when required.

Keep up a healthy lifestyle: The state of one's overall health and well-being affects the pelvic floor. Eat a balanced diet, remain hydrated, exercise often, control your stress levels and don't smoke. These elements may have a favourable effect on how well the pelvic floor muscles work.

It's crucial to speak with a healthcare provider if you have any questions or suffer symptoms connected to your pelvic floor so they can provide personalised advice and suggestions based on your particular requirements.

HOLISTIC APPROACHES TO FEMININE CARE

Diet and Nutrition for Feminine Health

In order to preserve feminine health, proper food and nutrition are quite important. A healthy diet that is well-balanced and comprehensive may assist to promote overall wellbeing, hormone balance, reproductive health and lower the risk of a number of health problems. Here are some food recommendations and nutrition advice designed especially for female health:

Diet: Make an effort to eat a varied selection of whole foods from each food category as part of a balanced diet. Fruits, vegetables, whole grains, lean meats and healthy fats should make up this diet.

Fibre-rich Foods: Include a lot of fibre-rich foods in your diet to promote digestive health and control bowel motions. Fruits, vegetables, whole grains, nuts and seeds all contain fibre.

Calcium and Vitamin D: These nutrients—calcium and vitamin D—are crucial for preserving bone health. Dairy products, leafy green vegetables and fortified plant-based milk are some examples of foods high in calcium. Sunlight exposure is the best way to get vitamin D, although it may also be gotten via supplements.

Iron-rich Foods: Foods high in iron help prevent anaemia, which is common in women and is more prevalent during menstruation. Red meat, chicken, fish, beans, lentils, tofu and fortified cereals are all excellent sources of iron.

Omega-3 Fatty Acids: These good fats are good for your heart, your brain, and your ability to fight inflammation. Fatty fish *(salmon, mackerel and sardines)*, chia seeds, flaxseeds and walnuts are sources of omega-3s.

Stay Hydrated: Drink enough water all day long to stay well hydrated and support your body's many functions.

Limit added sugars and Processed foods: Limit your intake of processed meals, sugary beverages and snacks since they may cause weight gain and have a detrimental effect on your general health.

Probiotics: Consume probiotic-rich foods like yoghurt, kefir, kimchi and sauerkraut to improve immune function and gastrointestinal health.

Healthy Fats: Include healthy fats from nuts, seeds, avocados, olive oil and other sources. These fats aid in the synthesis of hormones and the assimilation of fat-soluble vitamins.

Moderate Caffeine and Alcohol Intake: Limit your intake of coffee and alcohol, since too much of either may disturb hormone balance, impair sleep and generally be bad for your health.

Preventative Measures: Consuming cranberries or cranberry juice may help prevent urinary tract infections *(UTIs)*, and eating a balanced diet can help avoid a number of feminine health problems.

Consult a Healthcare expert: Individual dietary requirements might vary, therefore it's crucial to build a personalised nutrition plan that takes into account certain issues or conditions in consultation with a qualified dietitian or healthcare expert.

Folate and vitamin B12: For women of reproductive age, getting enough folate *(folic acid)* is essential because it helps prevent neural tube abnormalities in developing foetuses. Leafy greens, lentils, fortified cereals and citrus fruits are all excellent sources of folate. For the synthesis of red blood cells and normal neurological function, vitamin B12, which is predominantly found in animal products, is crucial. If you have a vegetarian or vegan diet, think about B12 pills or foods that have been fortified.

Phytoestrogens: Phytoestrogens are plant-based substances that have a weak estrogenic impact on the body. In certain women, they may help control hormonal equilibrium and lessen menopausal symptoms. Soy products, flaxseeds, chickpeas and lentils are all excellent sources.

Foods high in antioxidants: Antioxidants assist the body fend against oxidative damage and inflammation. To gain antioxidants like vitamin C, vitamin E, beta-carotene and selenium, include a range of vibrant fruits and vegetables in your diet.

Choline: For the liver and the health of the brain, choline is crucial. Eggs, liver, salmon and cruciferous vegetables like broccoli are excellent sources of choline.

Limited Sodium intake: Limit your salt consumption since it might cause bloating and in some people, elevate blood pressure. Choose fresh, natural meals that have been cooked with less salt added rather than processed and salty ones.

Maintain a Healthy Weight: Make an effort to keep your weight in check by eating a balanced diet and getting frequent exercise. Obesity and underweight both impair hormone balance and reproductive health.

Prevent Anaemia: Iron deficiency anaemia is more common in women than males, particularly during the menstrual cycle. By consuming meals high in vitamin C and foods high in iron, such as citrus fruits and spinach, you may improve your body's ability to absorb iron.

Keep an eye out for food intolerances and allergies: You should be aware of any dietary intolerances or allergies you may have as they might affect your general health and digestive system. Nuts, dairy and gluten are common allergies.

Preventative Health Screening: Gynaecological checks and screenings are important for preserving feminine health and spotting any possible problems early on. Preventative health screenings are also important.

Breast Health: A good diet and way of life may improve breast health in general, despite the fact that there are no particular foods that can prevent breast cancer. Conduct routine breast self-examinations and talk with your healthcare professional about screening possibilities.

Prenatal and Postnatal Nutrition: Work with a healthcare professional or qualified dietitian to ensure you're receiving the nutrients you need for a healthy pregnancy if you're pregnant or trying to conceive. After giving delivery, concentrate on eating a balanced diet to help breastfeeding and postnatal recovery.

Take Note of Your Body: Pay heed to your body's cues and act on them appropriately. Consult a healthcare provider right away if you encounter any unsettling signs or symptoms linked to your digestion, menstrual cycle or general health.

A healthy lifestyle includes much more than simply food and nutrition. Maintaining feminine health and general wellbeing requires regular exercise, stress reduction techniques and enough sleep.

Nourishing Foods for Hormonal Balance

For general health and wellbeing, maintaining hormonal balance is essential.
Here are some meals that might support hormonal balance:

Fatty Fish: Omega-3 fatty acids, which are abundant in fatty fish like salmon, mackerel and sardines, may aid to decrease inflammation and improve hormonal health.

Avocado: Avocados are an excellent source of monounsaturated fats, which are crucial for the generation of hormones.

Nuts and Seeds: Omega-3 fatty acids, fibre and protein, which may help regulate hormones, are found in nuts like almonds and walnuts as well as seeds like chia and flax seeds.

Leafy Greens: Dark leafy greens like spinach and kale are rich in minerals like magnesium, which may aid with hormone control.

Cruciferous Vegetables: Broccoli, cauliflower, Brussels sprouts and cabbage are cruciferous vegetables that contain indole-3-carbinol, which promotes the metabolism of oestrogen.

Berries: Antioxidants found in berries like blueberries, strawberries, and raspberries may fight oxidative stress and maintain hormonal balance in general.

Legumes: Beans, lentils and chickpeas are great sources of plant-based protein and fibre, which may help regulate blood sugar levels and maintain hormonal balance.

Foods High in Probiotics: Foods like yoghurt, kefir and fermented vegetables promote gut health, which is related to hormone balance.

Whole Grains: Whole grains like quinoa, brown rice, and oats provide complex carbs and fibre, which may promote hormonal balance and help keep blood sugar levels consistent.

Turmeric: Curcumin, an anti-inflammatory compound found in turmeric, may help hormonal balance.

Green Tea: Green tea is high in antioxidants and may improve insulin sensitivity and hormone balance.

Dark Chocolate: Consumed in moderation, dark chocolate may help lower levels of cortisol *(the stress hormone)* and elevate mood.

Healthy Fats: Incorporate sources of healthy fats like olive oil, coconut oil and grass-fed butter into your diet in addition to avocados and fatty seafood. These lipids are necessary for the development and control of hormones.

Manage Stress: Long-term stress may result in hormone abnormalities, especially high levels of cortisol. Practise stress-relieving methods like yoga, meditation, deep breathing or spending time in nature.

Regular Exercise: Exercise helps promote hormone balance and aid to increase insulin sensitivity. Find an activity you want to do and include it into your routine on a regular basis.

Avoid Endocrine Disruptors: Certain plastics, home cleansers and pesticides contain compounds that may disrupt hormone function. When feasible, choose for BPA-free goods, natural cleaning solutions and organic meals.

Balanced Meal Timing: Aim for frequent meals throughout the day and steer clear of excessive dieting or extended fasting, which may mess with your hormones' ability to produce and regulate them.

Quality of Sleep: Make obtaining enough restful sleep a top priority each night since insufficient sleep may have a detrimental influence on hormone levels and general health.

Check for dietary Sensitivity: Some people may have hormone imbalances as a result of certain dietary sensitivities. If you want to find and deal with any possible sensitivities, think about consulting with a healthcare expert.

Hormone-Supporting Herbs: Some plants, like chasteberry *(vitex)*, ashwagandha and maca root, have been used for centuries to maintain hormonal balance. Before including herbal supplements in your regimen, always seek medical advice.

Establishing hormonal balance is a complex process that includes making appropriate food choices, altering one's lifestyle, managing one's stress levels and taking care of any underlying medical conditions.

Nutrients for Optimal Vaginal Health

It's crucial for overall wellbeing to maintain excellent vaginal health. Although the vagina is a self-cleaning and self-regulating organ, certain foods and lifestyle choices may help to maintain its health. Consider the following essential vitamins and behaviours:

Probiotics are helpful bacteria that may keep the flora in the vagina in a healthy balance. Orally consumed supplements or fermented foods like yoghurt, kefir, kimchi and sauerkraut contain them. Probiotics help maintain a balanced pH in the vagina and lower the incidence of infections.

Vitamin D plays a crucial part in boosting the immune system. A healthy vaginal environment and infection prevention may be supported by adequate vitamin D levels. Vitamin D may be obtained via the sun, food sources including fatty fish and fortified dairy products or supplementation.

Vitamin C is an antioxidant that helps maintain the health of the vaginal and immune systems. It might help maintain a healthy vaginal pH level and lower the risk of certain infections. Excellent sources of vitamin C include citrus fruits, strawberries and leafy greens.

Zinc is necessary for immune system health and wound healing, both of which are advantageous in avoiding and treating vaginal infections. Red meat, whole grains, legumes, nuts, seeds and seeds are foods high in zinc.

Omega-3 fatty acids contain anti-inflammatory qualities that may help lessen vaginal tissue inflammation and promote overall vaginal health. Good sources of omega-3s include fatty fish, flaxseeds, chia seeds and walnuts. Also, It's essential for general health, especially vaginal health, to be hydrated. Consuming enough water may reduce pain and irritation while maintaining the moisture in the vagina.

Keep your vaginal region free of perfumed items, harsh washes and douches. These could cause discomfort or infections by upsetting the vaginal flora's normal equilibrium.

Even though the vagina is self-cleaning, keeping basic hygiene is still crucial. Use mild, scent-free soap and water to wash the external genital region. After using the restroom, always wipe from front to back to prevent bringing germs into the vaginal region.

Using condoms and engaging in safe sex might help avoid STIs that could harm vaginal health.

It's crucial to see your doctor often to check your vaginal health and treat any concerns or problems as soon as they arise.

Cranberry products: According to some research, cranberry pills or juice may help reduce urinary tract infections *(UTIs)*. Including cranberry products in your diet may be advantageous since UTIs may sometimes impact vaginal health.

By eliminating both dangerous and good bacteria, excessive or frequent antibiotic usage might upset the vaginal flora's delicate balance. Ask your doctor about measures to protect the health of your vagina during and after treatment if you require antibiotics for a bacterial infection.

Exercise promotes blood circulation, which may help maintain healthy vaginal tissues. Exercise is also good for general health. Exercise may also help you feel less stressed, which is important for your general health.

Excessive stress has a detrimental effect on the immune system and may be a factor in problems with vaginal health. Engage in stress-relieving activities like yoga, meditation, deep breathing exercises or enjoyable hobbies.

To promote airflow in the genital region, wear breathable, cotton pants. This may lessen the risk of infections by preventing the development of excessive moisture.

Do try to avoid too much sugar intake, it may lead to flora imbalances in the vagina, increasing the risk of infections. Limit your consumption of sweetened meals and drinks.

To lessen friction and pain if you feel vaginal dryness during sexual intercourse, think about using water-based lubricants. Avoid using silicone- or petroleum-based lubricants, since these may alter the pH of the vagina and cause discomfort.

Some birth control methods, such as some intrauterine devices *(IUDs)* or some kinds of oral contraceptives, might affect vaginal health. Discuss your worries with your healthcare practitioner if you see changes in your vaginal health after beginning or switching birth control methods.

Hormonal changes during perimenopause and menopause might have an impact on vaginal health. Dryness and soreness in the vagina are frequent at this period. Discuss possible medicines or treatments with your healthcare physician, such as vaginal moisturisers or oestrogen-based therapy.

Smoking should be avoided since it has a detrimental effect on the immune system and raises the risk of infection. Consider giving up smoking to improve your general health, which includes your vaginal health.

A variety of variables, including hormonal fluctuations, sexual activity and personal behaviours, might affect vaginal health. Consult a medical expert right away if you have chronic vaginal pain, an odd discharge or any other problems.

EXERCISE AND FITNESS FOR THE PELVIC FLOOR

Strengthening Pelvic Floor Muscles

Both men and women should strengthen their pelvic floor muscles since doing so may help prevent and treat a number of health concerns, including urine incontinence, pelvic organ prolapse and challenges with sexual function. Maintaining the strength of the pelvic floor muscles is essential for maintaining overall pelvic health since they support the bladder, uterus and bowel.

Here are some recommendations and exercises for building your pelvic floor muscles:

Kegel Exercises: The most popular and efficient exercise for strengthening the pelvic floor is the kegel. Follow these steps to do kegels:

- Recognise the pelvic floor muscles by attempting to halt the flow of urine midway the next time you pee. Your pelvic floor muscles are the ones you use for this.
- Once you've determined which muscles they are, empty your bladder and find a comfortable posture to sit or lay down in.
- Attempt to block the flow of pee or stop gas from flowing by contracting the muscles in your pelvic floor. These muscles should be tightened and held for 5 seconds.

Muscle Easing: After five seconds of respite, let go of the contraction.
Replicate the activity: Three times each day, aim for 10 to 15 repetitions.

Bridge Pose: Yoga's Bridge Pose improves the glutes and lower back in addition to the pelvic floor muscles.

- Legs bent and flat on the floor, hip-width apart, while you lay on your back.
- As soon as your body is in a straight line from your shoulders to your knees, lift your hips off the ground.
- During this action, contract your pelvic floor muscles and squeeze your glutes.
- After a little while, hold the position and then bring your hips back down.
- Repeat ten to fifteen times.

Squats: Squats work the muscles in your lower body and pelvic floor.

- Place your feet shoulder-width apart as you stand.
- Keep your back straight and your chest high as you lower your body as if you were sitting back into a chair.
- As you ascend back to the standing posture, contract the muscles in your pelvic floor.
- Do 10 to 15 repetitions.

Pilates: Pilates workouts often emphasise core strength, which includes the muscles of the pelvic floor.

Biofeedback: Some gadgets might provide biofeedback to assist you in accurately identifying and contracting your pelvic floor muscles.

Consistency: Like any fitness programme, persistence is essential to seeing results. Make pelvic floor exercises a part of your regular regimen.

Mind-Body Connection: Exercises for the pelvic floor need a strong mind-body connection, which must be developed. Without using any other muscle groups, concentrate on isolating and tightening the muscles in your pelvic floor. This control may take some time to master, but it is essential to the success of the workouts.

Breathing: The efficacy of pelvic floor exercises may be increased by using the right breathing methods. Deeply inhale while your pelvic floor muscles are relaxed and then exhale as you contract and elevate your pelvic floor muscles. Don't hold your breath when exercising.

Gradual Progression: If you're just starting off with pelvic floor exercises, start out gently and build up to a higher level of difficulty over time. As your muscles become stronger, start with shorter hold periods and fewer repetitions and work your way up.

Mix up the Exercises: Even though Kegels are the most popular pelvic floor exercises, it's important to vary your practice. To achieve healthy muscular growth, use a variety of workouts that target the pelvic floor from diverse angles.

Be patient; developing stronger pelvic floor muscles takes time. Significant progress could not be seen for weeks or even months. Be persistent and kind to yourself.

Body Posture: Maintain proper body alignment throughout the day. Try to stand and sit erect, avoiding slouching or hunching, since poor posture may strain the pelvic floor muscles.

Avoid High-Impact workouts: If you have pelvic floor problems, you should stay away from high-impact workouts since they may place additional pressure on the pelvic area. Running and leaping are two activities that might make certain disorders worse.

Maintain a Healthy Weight: Being overweight may add to the strain on the muscles of the pelvic floor, which may result in problems like urine incontinence. Pelvic health may benefit from maintaining a healthy weight with a balanced diet and frequent exercise.

Pelvic Floor Physical Therapy: Consider seeking the advice of a pelvic floor physical therapist if you are having problems with your pelvic floor, including discomfort or resistance to activity. They may provide you personalised advice, assess your pelvic floor muscles and recommend specially designed workouts to take care of your particular requirements.

Maintaining a healthy pelvic floor is important for individuals of all ages and genders. Pelvic floor exercises might be a preventative step for the future even if you aren't experiencing any problems right now.

Recommended Exercises and Techniques for Women

For the health of women, pelvic floor muscles must be strong and flexible. Here are some ways and exercises to maintain and develop the female pelvic floor:

Breathing exercises: Proper breathing methods may be used in conjunction with pelvic floor exercises to promote relaxation and better muscular control. To encourage ideal pelvic floor function, engage in belly breathing, sometimes referred to as diaphragmatic breathing.

- Choose a comfortable posture to sit or to lay down.
- Your chest and abdomen should be touched with one hand each.
- Allow your belly to expand as you inhale deeply through your nose.
- As you gently exhale out of your mouth, your stomach should compress.
- During exercises, pay attention to breathing in time with the contraction of your pelvic floor muscles.

Yoga: A lot of yoga positions involve relaxing and engaging the pelvic floor. Poses like "Cobra," "Child's Pose," and "Malasana" may assist the pelvic floor muscles to become stronger and more flexible.

Avoid high-impact workouts: If your pelvic floor is already weak, certain high-impact exercises, like leaping or sprinting, might place too much pressure on it. Consider low-impact workouts like swimming or cycling as alternatives if you have pelvic floor problems.

Core activities that are safe for the pelvic floor: Conventional core workouts like crunches may strain the pelvic floor. Instead, choose exercises that are good for your pelvic floor, such the "Dead Bug" or "Heel Slides."

Healthy living for the pelvic floor: In addition to exercise, leading a healthy lifestyle has benefits for the pelvic floor. To maintain a healthy pelvic floor, one should drink enough water, eat a diet high in fibre and keep a healthy weight.

Use relaxation techniques: Pelvic floor problems may be exacerbated by ongoing stress and tension. To reduce stress and encourage pelvic floor relaxation, try using relaxation methods like progressive muscle relaxation, tai chi, or meditation.

Postpartum pelvic floor care: After giving delivery, the pelvic floor has to be taken care of. Under the supervision of a healthcare practitioner, start off slowly and improve your pelvic floor exercises as your body recovers.

Regular check-ups: It's a good idea to see your doctor for periodic pelvic examinations and check-ups. Your pelvic floor's condition may be evaluated and any problems or concerns can be resolved.

Pelvic floor-friendly footwear: Regularly wearing high heels might damage your posture and the alignment of your pelvic floor. Choose supportive, comfortable footwear that encourages appropriate body alignment and posture.

Avoid prolonged sitting: Avoid sitting for extended periods of time since it might strain your pelvic floor. If your daily routine requires prolonged sitting, attempt to take pauses and engage in some light stretching or walking.

Pelvic floor awareness during daily activities: Being conscious of your pelvic floor muscles when doing everyday tasks such as moving heavy things, sneezing, laughing or coughing is important. During these times, engaging the pelvic floor may increase support and lessen strain.

Hydration and Bladder health: Keep yourself well hydrated to preserve the health of your bladder. However, limit your intake of coffee and alcohol since they might irritate your bladder and make you urinate more often.

Sexual activities that are safe for the pelvic floor: If you are worried about the health of your pelvic floor during sexual activity, look into postures and activities that are easier on the pelvic floor. A calm frame of mind and open conversation with your partner may also enhance your sexual experience.

Manage chronic coughing: Controlling persistent coughing is important because it might strain the pelvic floor. To treat the underlying cause of a chronic cough, seek medical help.

Techniques for bowel movements: Refrain from straining during bowel movements since this might weaken the pelvic floor and increase the risk of haemorrhoids and protrusion of the pelvic organs. Make sure you have enough time to go to the bathroom and keep a calm position on the toilet.

Manage your stress and anxiety: High levels of stress and worry may cause tightness and dysfunction in the pelvic floor. Take part in stress-relieving activities like deep breathing exercises, meditation or enjoyable hobbies.

Pelvic floor support devices: Your healthcare professional may sometimes advise using pessaries or other pelvic floor support devices to assist treat certain pelvic floor issues.

Pelvic floor education: Learn about the functions of the pelvic floor by doing some research on it. You can better take care of this vital component of your body if you know how the muscles function and what variables might affect their health.

Every woman's pelvic floor is different and some may have particular issues or disorders that call for specialised treatment. Consult a medical expert, particularly one who specialises in women's health or pelvic floor physical therapy, if you suffer any pelvic floor dysfunction symptoms, such as urine incontinence, pelvic discomfort or trouble pooping.

Lastly, when it comes to pelvic floor exercises, consistency is crucial. Be patient and incorporate these habits into your everyday routine since it can take some time before you see any changes. Keep up your commitment to preserving pelvic floor health since it may significantly improve your general wellbeing and quality of life.

FEMININE CARE: STRESS MANAGEMENT AND EMOTIONAL WELL-BEING

Women's total health and wellbeing includes factors including feminised care, stress management, and emotional stability. Let's examine each subject in turn:

Feminine Care:

The procedures and supplies used to keep a woman's private parts clean and healthy are referred to as feminine care. To avoid infections, maintain pH balance and foster comfort and confidence, proper feminine care is crucial.

These are some essential components of feminine care:

- **Individual Hygiene:** Wash your genital region with water and mild soap on a regular basis. Avoid using strong chemicals or douches since they might disturb the vagina's natural balance and raise the possibility of infections.

- **Menstrual Hygiene:** Use appropriate menstrual products, such as pads, tampons or menstrual cups, throughout your period to maintain good menstrual hygiene. To stop the formation of germs and subsequent illnesses, replace them often.

- Choose cotton pants that are breathable to promote airflow and prevent sweat from condensing in your undergarments.

- After sexual activity, urinate to help avoid urinary tract infections (UTIs).

- Gynaecological screenings and check-ups should be scheduled on a regular basis to monitor your reproductive health and treat any issues.

Stress Management: Although stress is a normal reaction to demanding or difficult circumstances, prolonged stress may have a detrimental influence on both physical and mental health.

Here are some methods for properly managing stress:

Exercise: Exercise often to produce endorphins that may aid with stress relief and mood improvement.

Meditation and Mindfulness: The mind may be calmed and relaxation can be encouraged by using practices like mindfulness and meditation.

Breathing Exercise: Deep breathing exercises may help the body relax and lower tension by triggering this reaction.

Time management: To prevent feeling overburdened, prioritise and organise your everyday chores.

Seek Support: If you are feeling a lot of stress or worry, seek support by talking to friends, family, or a therapist.

Hobbies and recreation: Take part in the pursuits you love to distract yourself from tensions and improve your general wellbeing.

Emotional Well-being:

Your capacity to manage your emotions, have a happy attitude and develop resilience is referred to as your emotional well-being.

Here are some pointers for improving emotional health:

Self-awareness: Pay attention to your sentiments and look for situations or people that might act as triggers for bad sensations.

Don't Suppress Your feelings: Find constructive methods to let your feelings out, such as speaking to a supportive friend or keeping a notebook.

Healthy Boundaries: To avoid emotional weariness in relationships, establish and maintain appropriate limits.

Social connection: Develop deep social ties with loved ones, friends or support networks to overcome feelings of loneliness.

Practice gratitude: Express your thanks for the good things in your life on a regular basis. This might help you feel happier overall.

Seek help if needed: When in doubt, ask for help from a mental health expert. If you're having trouble with your emotional stability.

Self-Compassion: Developing self-compassion is essential for maintaining emotional health. Be patient and understanding with yourself, even when things are difficult. You should show yourself the same compassion you would a buddy who was struggling. Recognise that everyone makes errors and that setbacks are to be expected. Focus on gaining from these experiences rather than being excessively critical.

Sleep hygiene: Getting enough sleep is crucial for both your physical and mental health. Set up a regular sleep pattern with a goal of 7-9 hours of good sleep each night. To tell your body it's time to wind down, establish a calming sleep ritual. Reduce screen time before bed since the blue light from electronics might interfere with sleep cycles.

Nutrition: Emotional health is a component of total well-being, which is enhanced by eating a balanced diet. A mix of fruits, vegetables, whole grains, lean proteins and healthy fats should be consumed. As even little dehydration may impact mood and cognitive performance, stay hydrated all day long.

Activities that Help decrease tension: Take part in activities that help decrease tension and encourage relaxation. Reading, being outside, taking warm baths, doing yoga or listening to peaceful music are some examples of this. Make time for the things you like on a regular basis.

Setting Healthy Boundaries and Saying No: Develop the ability to say no when it's called for. Stress and emotional strain may develop when people take on too many obligations or feel pressure to impress others. Knowing when to turn down more obligations and when to prioritise self-care can help you prioritise your well-being.

Professional Support: If you're having trouble coping with stress, emotional difficulties, or old traumas, you may want to think about getting help from a therapist or counsellor. Speaking with a mental health expert may provide insightful advice, coping mechanisms and a secure environment in which to work through emotional problems.

Community and Support Networks: Find others who share your interests or join support groups that cover the issues that are bothering you. A feeling of communal support may provide people a sense of understanding and belonging, which supports emotional health.

A woman's physical health, stress management and emotional wellness must all be maintained for her overall health and happiness. Quality of life may be greatly enhanced and you can overcome obstacles in life with more resilience by implementing self-care practices, asking for assistance when you need it and adopting good lifestyle choices.

THE MIND-BODY CONNECTION

A key component of holistic health and wellbeing is the idea of the mind-body link. It acknowledges the complex interactions between and influences on one another of both mental and bodily states. Nurturing this connection becomes crucial for fostering general health, self-assurance and empowerment when it comes to feminine intimate care.

A variety of procedures are included in feminine intimate care with the goal of keeping a woman's genital region clean and healthy. The effects of these practices on the mind cannot be understated, even if they entail physical components like washing, moisturising and using the right products.

Female personal care may, first and foremost, promote a strong feeling of self-awareness. Women may strengthen their bond with themselves by paying attention to this often underappreciated body area. As a result of their increased awareness, they may spot any changes or irregularities that would need medical treatment, leading to the early identification and avoidance of any health problems.

Regular intimate care routines may also be a way to take care of and love oneself. By taking the time to care for one's intimate region, one may foster a healthy connection with their body and develop an understanding of their own requirements. This supportive feedback may aid in overcoming cultural pressures and erroneous beauty standards that often result in body image problems and anxieties.

Using feminine intimate care techniques might help you unwind and decompress. These rituals, like other self-care practices like meditation or yoga, may be implemented into a daily or weekly schedule to bring about a moment of serenity. Women who take the time to pamper and care for themselves experience less stress and worry, which results in a general improvement in their mental health.

The mind-body connection may be further strengthened by the items used in feminine intimate care. The danger of irritation may be reduced and a careful approach to this delicate region can be ensured by using natural, organic, and chemical-free products. The delicate aromas and textures of these goods may have a calming impact on the mind, fostering a sense of comfort and wellbeing.

Relationships and sexual health may benefit from developing a healthy mind-body connection via intimate care practices. A healthy sexual self-image results in more closeness and communication with partners. Feeling secure and at ease with one's body is a factor in this. A meaningful and pleasant personal life may be created by this good energy, which can also raise the general quality of relationships.

It is important to keep in mind that every woman's body is different, and what works for one woman may not work for another. When choosing products and establishing personal care routines, individual preferences, sensitivities, and health concerns should always be taken into account. A specialist's or healthcare professional's consultation may provide insightful advice suited to your unique requirements and circumstances.

Accepting the mind-body link in feminine intimate care may result in a significant change in how society views and values women's bodies. Intimate care-related conversations have traditionally been veiled in shame and secrecy, fostering an environment of discomfort and avoidance.

Women may fight these antiquated beliefs and open the door to a more tolerant and inclusive society by publicly recognising and prioritising feminine intimate care as an essential component of overall health.

In this shift, empowerment is essential. Women become active participants in their well-being when they feel empowered to manage their intimate care. When people feel empowered, they are more likely to speak up for their rights, make wise choices about their bodies and promote improved healthcare. Intimate care practices that strengthen the mind-body link may encourage resilience, bravery and assertiveness, empowering women to face obstacles head-on.

The mind-body link may have an effect on the immune system and general physical health in the context of holistic health. Chronic stress and unfavourable emotions have been found in studies to damage the immune system, leaving the body more vulnerable to disease. Through intimate care rituals, women may boost their immune systems and enhance their general health and well-being by encouraging relaxation, uplifting feelings and self-care.

Additionally, using mindfulness techniques while doing intimate care rituals may improve the experience and strengthen the mind-body connection. Being completely present in the moment and paying attention to one's thoughts, emotions and physical sensations without passing judgement on them are both aspects of mindfulness.

Women who practise mindfulness while doing intimate care get a better comprehension of their bodies' needs and reactions, which enables them to recognise any pain or problems that may need to be addressed.

The release of stress and unfavourable feelings that may have been held in the pelvic region is another benefit of using mindfulness into intimate care.

A feeling of emotional liberation and healing may be facilitated by thoughtful self-care, which can help relieve the tension and trauma that many women hold in this area of the body.

Fostering the mind-body link in feminine intimate care requires open communication and education. It's essential to remove the stigma associated with talking about women's personal health in order to ensure that appropriate information is shared.

Women are better able to make educated decisions, ask for assistance when necessary, and recognise the importance of their intimate health for their overall wellbeing when open communication is encouraged.

In terms of feminine intimate care, the mind-body link is a potent and transformational idea that goes beyond physical health. Women may enhance their emotional, mental and sexual health by fostering this connection, which helps them become more self-aware, self-confident and empowered. Embracing personal care as a crucial component of self-care enables women to defy social expectations and fight for their rights and overall well being.

Women may relieve mental stress, boost their immune systems and develop a healthy connection with their bodies via mindfulness and knowledge. A path of self-discovery, acceptance and empowerment, recognising the mind-body link in feminine intimate care may have a significant and long-lasting influence on women's life.

STRATEGIES FOR STRESS REDUCTION

For general well-being, even when it comes to feminine intimate care, stress reduction is crucial. The health of the reproductive system is one of the many physical and mental effects of stress. Here are some stress-reduction techniques that are particularly geared towards feminine intimate care:

- Stress reduction and mental calming are two benefits of these practices. Regular practice may increase your capacity for stress management and foster a feeling of inner serenity.

- Endorphins, or "feel-good" hormones, are released during physical exercise such as yoga, swimming, or even brisk walking, which may help lower stress. Additionally, exercise increases blood flow, which is advantageous for sexual health.

- Using deep breathing methods will help the body relax and lower stress levels. Whenever you feel worried or overwhelmed, practise taking calm, deep breaths.

- Make sleep a priority by making sure you receive adequate sound sleep every night. The reproductive system as well as the body's healing and recovery functions depend on sleep.

- Setting limits in both your personal and professional lives might help you feel less stressed. It's important to prioritise self-care and set aside time for yourself.

- Don't be reluctant to discuss your thoughts and worries with a dependable friend, member of your family or a therapist. Pent-up tension and emotions may be released via self-expression.

- Find relaxing things you like doing, such as reading, listening to music, taking a bath or spending time in nature.

- Recognise the stressors in your life and work to reduce your exposure to them. This can be minimising the amount of time spent on social media, avoiding upsetting news or better time management.

- To lessen the chance of itchiness or pain, use feminine care products that are manufactured with natural and mild components. Be cautious of strong scents and chemicals that could disturb the intimate area's natural equilibrium.

- Regular check-ups and screenings with your doctor will help you address any health issues and provide you peace of mind.

- Having a healthy diet and drinking enough water will help you feel better overall, which can help you feel less stressed.

- Be kind and compassionate to yourself, particularly when you are dealing with difficulties or disappointments. Embrace self-compassion instead of self-criticism to strengthen your resistance to stress.

- Use your senses to relax and unwind by engaging in sensory relaxation. Use aromatherapy to relax with relaxing smells like lavender or chamomile, take a warm bath to unwind or reward yourself with a light massage.

- Reduce intake of coffee and alcohol since both might make you feel more stressed and anxious. Limiting these drugs may make you feel more at ease and enhance the quality of your sleep.

- Establishing and sustaining healthy connections may provide emotional support and a feeling of community, both of which are good for lowering stress.

- A number of herbal teas, including chamomile, passionflower and peppermint, offer relaxing characteristics that may help reduce tension and encourage relaxation.

- Writing down your thoughts, emotions and experiences in a journal may help you process your feelings and gain perspective on difficult circumstances.

- Laughter is a great stress reliever. Spend time with those who make you laugh, watch a funny movie, or read a hilarious book.

- Look into holistic practices that are thought to promote stress reduction and general wellbeing, such as acupuncture, acupressure or reflexology.

- To prevent overstimulation and promote mental relaxation, take breaks from electronic devices and social media.

- Break projects down into small chunks and establish reasonable objectives for yourself. Feelings of tension and overload may be lessened by using this strategy.

- Focusing on the good parts of your life on a regular basis will help you avoid stress and enhance your attitude.

- Don't be afraid to seek assistance from a mental health professional or counsellor who specialises in stress management if stress is seriously affecting your everyday life.

- Finding a healthy way to release stress may be as simple as painting, writing or playing an instrument.

- Use the progressive muscle relaxation method to relax and relieve physical stress by tensing and then relaxing various muscle groups.

During menstruation or other periods of pelvic stress, using a warm compress or heating pad on your lower abdomen may help soothe sore muscles and reduce pain. Also pelvic floor exercises should be performed since they may enhance blood flow to the reproductive system and strengthen the muscles that support it. Additionally helpful in stress management are strong pelvic muscles.

- Some essential oils, such as rose, ylang-ylang and clary sage, have been linked to stress relief and relaxation. Use diluted essential oils for aromatherapy massage or in a diffuser.

- Practise progressive muscle relaxation for pelvic muscles, using this method, which is similar to progressive muscle relaxation, you deliberately tense and relax your pelvic muscles to relieve stress and tension.

Learn About Feminine Intimate Care:

Having knowledge about reproductive health and feminine intimate care will help you make wise choices and lessen your concern about these issues. Water-based or silicone-based lubricants, which are devoid of harsh chemicals, may be used to increase comfort and minimise friction during sexual activity.

Spend time sensually interacting with your body and discovering what makes you feel comfortable and happy. Self-care that is sensuous may lower stress and increase body confidence. Less sugary and processed foods will help to improve your hormonal balance and general wellbeing.

Practising Tai Chi or Qigong can help you unwind, relieve tension and increase your energy flow. These ancient arts blend movement, breathing and meditation. Most importantly maintaining excellent cleanliness will help prevent irritation and maintain a healthy vaginal environment. *Examples of good hygiene habits include* donning breathable pants, avoiding douching and quickly changing out of damp garments.

To tell your body it's time to relax, create a tranquil bedtime routine. This might be doing light stretches, reading a book or sipping herbal tea.

Volunteering or giving back may reduce stress and foster emotional well-being. It can also give one a feeling of fulfilment and purpose. Engaging in "forest bathing", nature-based activities, particularly in lush green settings, may have a relaxing impact on the body and mind.

Practise Emotional Release by giving yourself permission to openly express your feelings by sobbing, yelling or participating in expressive art. Do not subject yourself to undue pressure to achieve perfection. Accept your flaws and remember that it's OK to pause, regroup and seek assistance.

Never forget how important it is to pay attention to your needs and to your body. Be patient with yourself as you experiment with various techniques and discover which ones work best for you since everyone's road towards stress reduction is different. You may have a good influence on your overall health and feminine intimate care by giving stress management and self-care first priority.

SELF-CARE AND EMOTIONAL SUPPORT

Maintaining general wellbeing and mental health requires both self-care and emotional support. In order to manage stress, avoid burnout, and encourage a healthy, balanced lifestyle, they comprise practices and tactics aimed at caring for oneself on a physical and emotional level. *The following are important components of self-care and emotional support:*

Taking care of your physical health is an essential component of self-care. This includes obtaining adequate rest, maintaining a healthy diet, exercising often and taking care of any medical requirements.

Practices like mindfulness and meditation may help you remain present and focused, lower your stress levels and develop your self-awareness. It fosters a feeling of peace and clarity by allowing you to examine your thoughts and emotions without passing judgement.

Having strong bonds with friends, family, and other loved ones is essential for providing emotional support. Spending time with loved ones and participating in social activities may provide comfort and a feeling of belonging.

Setting Clear Boundaries and Learning to Say "No": Important elements of self-care include learning to say "no" when required and setting clear boundaries. It aids in keeping you from taking on too much and being stressed.

Effective time management may lower stress and boost productivity, freeing up more time for self-care activities and emotional well-being. Avoid self-criticism and practise self-compassion by being nice to oneself.

To counteract negative ideas and develop a more optimistic outlook, use positive affirmations. Journaling may be a useful tool for tracking progress, processing emotions, and understanding your own ideas and feelings.

Recognise sources of stress in your life and take action to reduce or successfully manage them and take pauses from social media and technological gadgets to clear your mind and encourage relaxation.

Nature and the outdoors: Being outside and taking part in outdoor activities may help to relax and rejuvenate the body and mind.

Laughter & Humour: Add some humour to your life by watching comedic television, reading jokes or hanging out with others who make you laugh. Laughter may be a wonderful stress reliever and mood booster.

Practise letting go of circumstances or concerns that you cannot alter and acknowledge that there are things that are out of your control. Put all of your efforts into what you can manage.

Volunteering and Kindness: Performing acts of kindness and helping others may make you feel fulfilled and give your life a sense of direction. Set aside some time each day to consider your blessings. This easy technique might help you turn your attention to the good things in your life.

Deep breathing exercises or mindfulness practices might help you when you're feeling anxious or overwhelmed. You may feel more at ease and relaxed as a result of it.

Hugging and Physical Contact: Physical contact, such as hugging, causes the release of oxytocin, a hormone that fosters emotions of closeness and lowers stress.

Limiting Negative Influences: Be careful who you associate with and what media you see. Limit your exposure to harmful influences that might harm your mental health. Always appreciate your successes, no matter how minor, since they will boost your motivation and self-esteem.

Create a Calming Environment: Plan an area in your house or place of business that encourages calmness and relaxation so you may rest and rejuvenate and to give oneself a feeling of purpose and success, set attainable objectives for both the short term and the long term.

Rekindle pastimes or passions you once loved but may have neglected. Taking part in these pursuits may be enjoyable and fulfilling.

Schedule time to routinely check in with yourself. Consider your feelings, requirements and self-care practices. Make use of self-help literature, apps or online forums that emphasise self-care and emotional well-being.

Take Mental Health Days: Don't be afraid to take a day off from work or other obligations if you're feeling overburdened or emotionally spent in order to recharge.

Use the progressive muscle relaxation method to alleviate physical tension and encourage relaxation by tensing and relaxing various muscle groups.

Experimenting and moving outside of your comfort zone may be energising and fulfilling for your mental wellbeing.

Reflect on your emotions, actions and patterns often to improve understanding of your emotional requirements and potential growth areas.

Investigate nature therapy: Spend time in environments that are naturally peaceful and tranquil, such as parks, woods, or the beach.

Practise Self-Compassion When You Facing Setbacks: When you encounter difficulties or setbacks, be kind to yourself. You should be nice to yourself as you would a good friend.

Limit multitasking to improve productivity and lessen stress. Concentrate on one activity at a time

Keep up with current events, but limit your exposure to upsetting news, particularly before night. Use visualisation methods to practise imagining favourable outcomes and lowering worry about upcoming occurrences.

Exercise produces endorphins, which may elevate mood and lessen stress, also give yourself some alone time to think, rejuvenate and do things by yourself that you like.

Avoid Abusing Substances: Drugs and alcohol may make emotional problems worse, so refrain from using them as a coping mechanism.

The goals of self-care and emotional support are to respect and care for you. It's not self-serving; rather, it's essential for your general wellbeing. As you adopt these habits into your life, have patience with yourself.

CONCLUSION:

Embracing Feminine Intimate Care

Accepting feminine intimate care is understanding how crucial it is to protect and preserve the health and wellbeing of the female reproductive system. It includes a range of behaviours, items and practises that promote comfort, hygienic conditions, and general vaginal health. Embracing feminine intimate care involves the following important factors:

Cleanliness: Maintaining good vaginal health requires proper cleanliness. This includes using mild, unscented soap or water for delicate cleaning. Use of strong chemicals, douches or scented items should be avoided since they might disturb the pH balance naturally and cause irritation or infections.

Menstrual care: It's important to use sanitary items like pads, tampons, or menstrual cups while you're menstruating. These products must be changed often to stop bacterial development and lower the risk of illnesses.

Be careful while selecting the things you use in and around your private areas. Avoid wearing clothing that is too tight since it might trap sweat and cause discomfort or infections. Instead, use breathable fabrics like cotton. Look for products with gentle, natural ingredients and without strong chemicals or smells when using items like wipes or washes made exclusively for intimate care.

Visits to a gynaecologist on a regular basis are necessary for maintaining excellent reproductive health. These examinations may aid in spotting problems early on and guarantee fast treatment if required.

Take care of your sexual health and safety in addition to embracing feminine intimate care. Sexually transmitted diseases *(STIs)* may be avoided by using protection, such as condoms and by being honest with your partner about your sexual health.

A balanced diet and enough water are important for general health, which includes vaginal health. Your body's immune system may be supported and infections can be avoided by drinking adequate water and eating a nutritious, well-balanced diet.

Kegel exercises: Kegel exercises may help to preserve bladder and bowel control as well as sexual enjoyment by strengthening the pelvic floor muscles.

Emotional well-being: An important component of general well-being, including interpersonal care, is acknowledging and managing emotional and mental health. Indirectly, the hormonal balance and vaginal health may be affected by stress and worry.

Recognising your body: Know the patterns of your vaginal discharge, your menstrual cycle, and any potential alterations or anomalies. Your self-awareness will enable you to see any possible health issues at an early stage.

Getting expert advice: Consult a medical practitioner if you encounter any unexpected symptoms, pain, or changes in your intimate region. If necessary, they can provide a precise diagnosis and the right treatment.

Feminine intimate care is about educating yourself, accepting your body's normal functions and forming healthy routines to promote your wellbeing. Every woman has a different physique, what works for one woman may not work for another. Make decisions based on your body's signals and your unique demands.

So Ladies, let's stay Clean, Fresh and Empowered

You can also check out our women's health publication

Low Sugar Diet For FIBROIDS & HORMONAL IMBALANCE

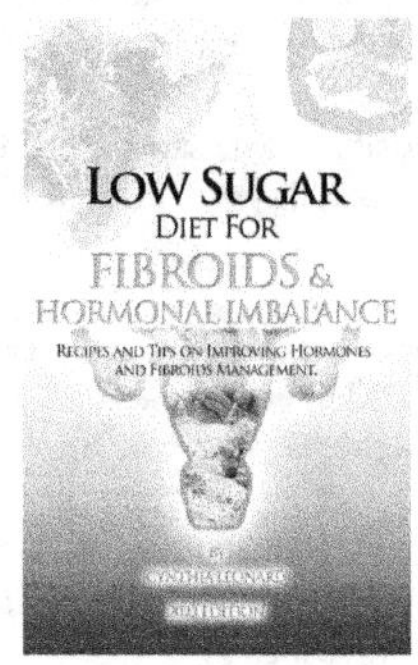